Fundamental Notions of

Endocrinology and Criminology

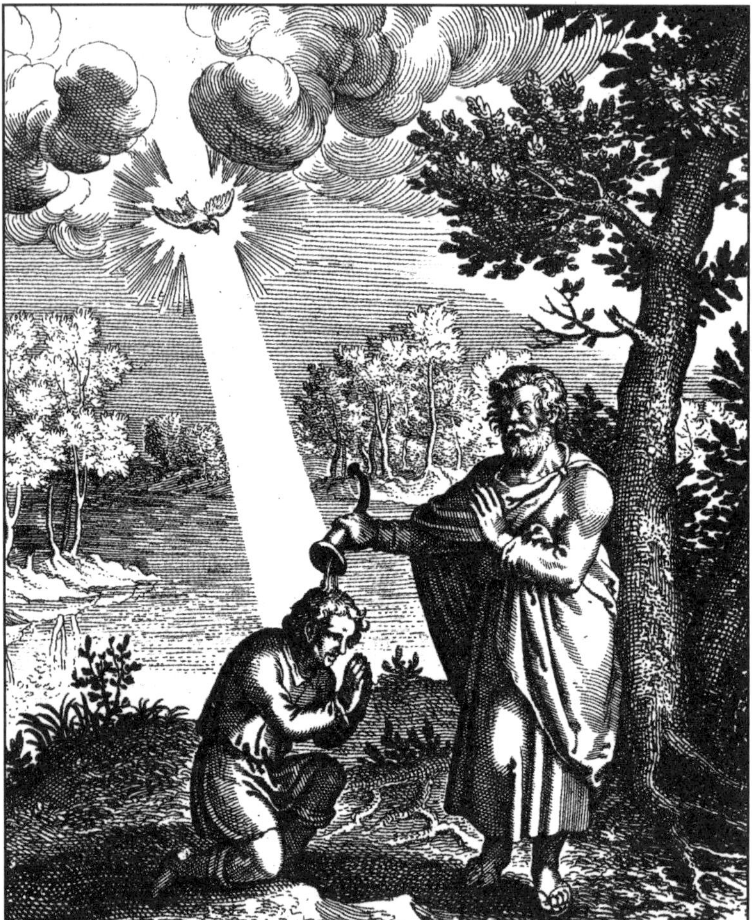

Baptism, the sacred symbol of Alchemy

Blessed be God, who has created Mercury,
because without it, the great work would
not be possible for the Alchemists.

Fundamental Notions of Endocrinology and Criminology

Gnosis, Practical Alchemy, Criminal Justice and Clairvoyance

Samael Aun Weor

Thelema Press
2007

Fundamental Notions of Endocrinology and Criminology
A Thelema Press Book / 2007

Originally published as "Nociones Fundamentales de Endocrinologia y Criminologia," 1959

ISBN: 978-1-934206-11-9

Thelema Press is a non-profit organization delivering to humanity the teachings of Samael Aun Weor. All proceeds go to further the distribution of these books. For more information, visit our website.

www.gnosticteachings.org
www.gnosticradio.org
www.gnosticschool.org
www.gnosticstore.org
www.gnosticvideos.org

Contents

Introduction

The Seven Planets of Alchemy

Although it may appear to be incredible, it is true and factually certain that the science of endocrinology is closely related to Sexual Alchemy. Endocrinology is bound to produce a true creative revolution. Scientists already know that the sexual glands are not sealed capsules. The sexual glands absorb and secrete hormones. The hormones of secretion are called "conserving," because they perpetuate the species. The hormones of absorption are called "vitalizing," because they vitalize the human organism. This process of hormonal absorption is transmutation; it is Alchemy: the transformation of one type of energy-matter into another type of energy-matter.

Sexual Magic is intensified sexual transmutation. Through Sexual Alchemy, the alchemist absorbs, transmutes and sublimates the totality of the sexual energy-matter. The rich and abundant sexual hormones inundate the circulatory system of the blood and reach the different glands of internal secretion, stimulating and inciting our endocrine system to work intensely. Thus, with intensified sexual transmutation, the endocrine glands are super-stimulated, naturally producing a greater number of hormones that animate and modify the entire fluid nervous system.

As the planets of our solar system revolve harmoniously around the Sun, likewise the different glands of our internal secretion harmoniously revolve throughout our blood. This is how our glands hormonally and harmoniously stimulate and incite our metabolism to work intensely.

Endocrinology, studied through Alchemy, enters into the fields of psychology and astrology. When the endocrine glands are super-stimulated, they naturally produce a greater number of hormones that animate the metallic (hormonal) planets of Alchemy within us.

If we see the order of the planets in a clear and Alchemical manner, we can then draw a perfect schematic diagram.

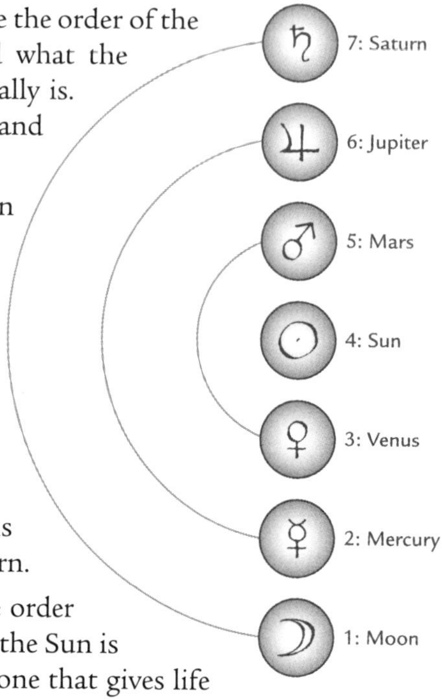

Observe carefully. Observe the order of the planets to try to understand what the work of Sexual Alchemy actually is. In front of us we have Saturn, and below us we have the Moon.

Let us now establish an Alchemical order of the planets: above the Moon is Mercury; a little above that is Venus; then the king of the sky, the Sun; Mars, the planet of war is further up; then we continue with Jupiter, and immediately after that, as I have already stated, is the most elevated planet, Saturn.

If we carefully observe the order of the planets, we can see that the Sun is in the center. The Sun is the one that gives life to all of the planets of the solar system.

One can achieve marvelous transformations through Sexual Alchemy. As we study Alchemy, it is necessary to know that these planets have their exponents in our own seminal system and within our own physical organism here and now.

Within us, through Sexual Alchemy, Saturn, the Ancient of the heavens, converts itself into the Moon. Why? Because the two extremes mutually correspond to each other.

Through Sexual Alchemy, Jupiter, which represents our innermost Being, is transformed into Mercury (of the secret philosophy). For one to see his own Mercury before the mirror of Alchemy, is precisely the most interesting part of this great astrological, psychological, and endocrine work. According to the great sages, this is when our own particular psychological Saint Thomas (which each person carries within) becomes confused and bewildered.

Therefore, Jupiter transformed into Mercury is something extraordinary. It is then that the Astral Body splendidly bursts forth, producing a magnificent change in our psyche.

Mars should be converted into Venus. That belligerent and terrible Mars that warrior and fighter that each of us carries within our depths should be transformed into the Venus of love.

Finally, it is the Sun that remains at the center, giving life to our entire inner psychic constitution. Therefore, those metallic planets are also found within our own metallic chaos. This metallic chaos is our seminal system, the Ens Seminis (entity of the semen).

It is astonishing indeed that venerable old Saturn is transformed and converted into a child of captivating beauty. This child has to be born within us. As the psychiatrists state, each person in his old age becomes a child, is converted into a child.

It is extraordinary that through Sexual Alchemy, thundering Jupiter, whose wife is Hera, the symbolic Sacred Cow, Devi Kundalini Shakti, the very essence of our sexual matter, is converted into the Mercury of the secret philosophy, into that Mercury that we come to see through the extraordinary mirror of Alchemy.

The great masters of Alchemy have stated:

> *Blessed be God, who has created Mercury, because without it, the great work would not be possible for the Alchemists.*

Mercury indeed astonishes us. Mercury is derived from the sexual hormonal transmutations, the transformations of the sacred sperm. Mercury is the outcome of Sexual Magic. It is like the vapor that rises from the will, like the cloud that rises from the metallic chaos.

This Mercury, however, possesses a sublime, ineffable type of intelligence. Indeed, this is how the lead of our personality can be transformed into that magnificent spiritual gold. Mercury can also be shown through our face. Mercury can be seen through the mirror of Alchemy.

If we think of Mars, the warrior, the Lord of Iron, if we think of those bellicose forces that we carry within our interior, if we think of those hard and terrible forces, we cannot but be astonished to see how, through Sexual Alchemy, they are transformed into the Lord of Love. This is how the Lord of Love is born in us.

This invites us to meditate on how the venerable Ancient of the Centuries converts himself into the child of affection that moves himself within the temples of the Universal White Fraternity.

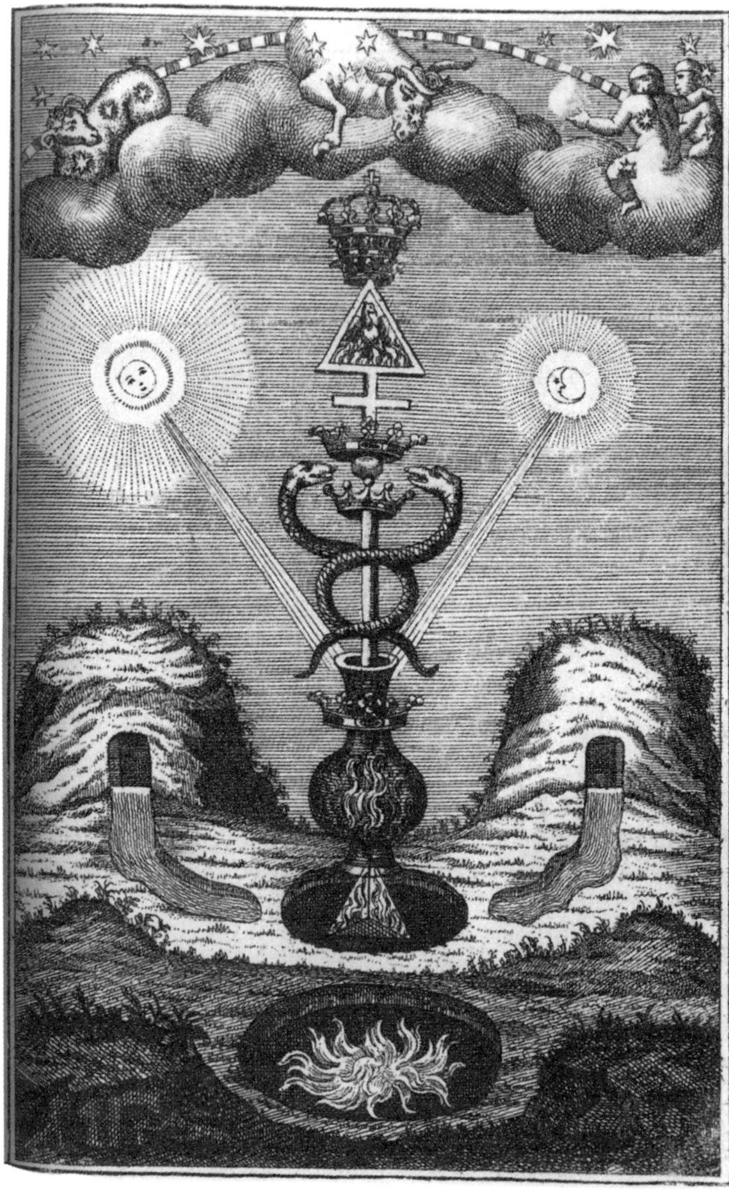

Mercurial Diagram by A.T. de Limojon de Saint-Didier, from Le Triomphe hermétique, 1689.

The Alchemist is bewildered, amazed, when thundering Jupiter, this ineffable Third Logos, this Arch-hierophant and Arch-magician of which the famous Spanish writer Mr. Mario Roso de Luna speaks, is transformed into the Mercury of occult philosophy, into the God of Eloquence.

The Mercury of occult philosophy is transformed into that lucid form of Cagliostro or into the portentous form of St. Germain, or simply, into the apotheosis of our psyche during magnificent ecstasy. Indeed, this cannot but astonish us.

I, Samael Aun Weor, have been able to see my own Mercury reflected through the mirror of Alchemy. I give testimony of what I have seen, and indeed it is grandiose.

Mercury is not only the outcome of the transformations of the sperm into energy, and Mercury is not only the agent through which we are able to convert lead into gold. The last words about Mercury have not yet been said. The explanation about Mercury is complete when we state that this Mercury is more than a pure metallic agent capable of bringing about transmutations. There is something else in that Mercury, in that God of Eloquence, in that living genie who shines in the Astral Body of the Alchemist. Mercury, indeed, is the very Logos converted or transformed through Sexual Magic into the Son of Man.

Mercury is not, therefore, a mere gross substance, or merely metallic. It is not only that sacred material spoken of by Sendivogius, Raymond Lully, Nicholas Flamel, Paracelsus, Eltrevisano, etc., but Mercury is something more. Mercury is thundering Jupiter converted into a manifested genie, thundering Jupiter converted into the metallic planet of Mercury.

Metallically speaking, we can state that it is this status converted into that beautiful and perfect creature that wanders in the temples, among the Elder Friends of humanity.

It amazes us greatly, beloved reader, how Sexual Alchemy produces in us the permutations of the metallic planets, the transformations of the planets one into the other, the radical change that gives birth to a new transcendental psychological creature.

How can it be or in what manner can we cause these metallic permutations within ourselves? Obviously, without the sacred fire of Alchemy, without Sexual Magic, it would become impossible for us to make changes of this type.

As you are now realizing, dear reader, we are, through Sexual Alchemy, seeking to convert ourselves into something psychologically different, to become someone psycho-physiologically distinct. We attain it through the transmutation of the diverse chemical substances that are combined within our organism and are related with the diverse biomechanical or physiological functions of our endocrine glands. If so many catalytic and metabolic phenomena exist, if sugar can be transformed into alcohol, undoubtedly diverse Alchemical permutations can also exist. Indeed, these Alchemical permutations, through unending combinations, convert us into almighty, divine, and ineffable Beings. Obviously, the Sahaja Maithuna, Sexual Magic, is the living foundation of this Great Work.

Planetary Influences

The human being enters the maternal womb as a mere germinating seed to develop and evolve. After nine months, the same seed comes into existence more developed, but still not completely developed.

During the first seven years of childhood, we live under the lunar influence. We then enjoy the happiness of the home, unless some negative Karma harms these first years of our life. Yet, the seed is still not completely developed, it is still in the process of development.

The fact that a germinating seed has been born, that a child came into existence somewhat more developed, does not mean that this seed, this child, has finished its development.

During the first seven years of our existence, there becomes manifested in our organism, in the males, the first testicular layer that permits them to exist, and as to females, their ovaries produce certain cells, certain principles, that vitally sustain them.

Later, that seed, continuing its process of development, enters under the influence of Mercury. Then the child goes to school, studies, learns, plays, etc. The child can no longer remain at home at all times. Mercury moves him, agitates him, and makes him restless. The second testicular layer produces in the male particular cells that come to specify and to completely define his sex. The female's ovaries produce certain cells, certain principles, that come to specify and to completely define her sex.

Age	Common Humanity	Initiates
0 - 7	Moon	Moon
7 - 14	Mercury	Mercury
14 - 21	Venus	Venus
21 - 42	Sun	Sun
42 - 49	Mars	Mars
49 - 56	Jupiter	Jupiter
56 - 63	Saturn	Saturn
63 - 70	Saturn + Moon	Uranus
70 - 77	Saturn + Mercury	Neptune
77 - 84	Saturn + Venus	Pluto

Planetary Influences and Age

In our development between fourteen and twenty-one years of age, we pass under the influence of Venus. It is stated that this is the age of falling in love. Men and women begin to experience sexual restlessness, because the sexual glands become activated. The third testicular zone in the male develops and produces sperm, but the latter are still not sufficiently mature, because the male who is between fourteen and twenty-one years of age has not completed his process of development. The seed has not concluded its process of development.

Therefore, it is very serious that a seed, which has not finished its natural process of development, enters into the field of sexual commerce. Undoubtedly, sexual intercourse is not advisable for seeds that have not yet completed their development.

It is not proper for a male who is undergoing his second infancy or adolescence to copulate. It is obvious that copulation between seeds that have not completed their development, or in other words, by teenagers or adolescents, undoubtedly, irrefutably, seriously damages their physical and mental health.

These damages, if not felt during youth, are felt during old age. This is how and why it is normal today for a man to begin losing his virility between the ages of forty and fifty years old. Why? Because of the abuse in his adolescence and during his second childhood.

We have already stated that the first childhood is from birth to the age of seven and that the second childhood is between seven and fourteen years of age.

Unfortunately, although it is pitiful to realize it, nowadays many children of twelve and thirteen years of age are already copulating. Moreover, those who are not yet copulating commit the crime of masturbation. They eliminate their hormones, degenerate their brains and atrophy their pineal gland through masturbation. This is how they become sure candidates for a mental home.

It is well known that after coitus, the phallus continues with certain peristaltic movements conducive to receiving vital energies from the feminine uterus in an attempt to replace its wasted creative principles.

However, when masturbation exists, instead of assimilating vital feminine energies with such peristaltic movements, useful principles for existence, the masturbator absorbs cold air, which passes directly to the brain. The outcome of this is idiocy, mental degeneration or insanity.

The vice of masturbation is, unfortunately, also very popular among the feminine sex. Obviously, with such a vice, many women that could have been genial or good wives have prematurely become degenerated, have aged quickly, have lost their sexual potential, and have become true victims of life.

Therefore, it is important to know all these aspects of sex; it is important to know what sex is.

For adolescents to have sex is absurd, because they are mere seeds which have not yet completed their development.

Development, in itself and by itself, concludes at the age of twenty-one. That is when adulthood really begins, the "responsible age" as it has already been called.

It is between twenty-one and forty-two years of age that we have to conquer our place under the Sun. Our vocation, whatever we are to be, remains forever decided.

Unfortunately, those who have reached adulthood, ordinarily have not had a specific upright sexual education. They have squandered their hormone capital and wasted their virile potency without having completed their development as seeds that one day enter the maternal womb. Thus, on arriving at the age of twenty-one, they discover that they have very weak mental strength.

Obviously, the pineal gland and the sexual glands are intimately related. So, mental strength and mental force are radiated by the pineal gland. Yet, when this gland has been weakened by sexual abuses, then the outcome is that we are at a very disadvantageous position in trying to conquer our place under the Sun.

Consequently, when we are not capable to radiate our psychic waves with force due to the weakness of the pineal gland, located in the upper part of our brain, we fail professionally, or the labor for our daily bread becomes more difficult. Our business fails and those people with whom we should establish commercial ties do not feel our drive, cancel their business with us and we are then hardly able to obtain our daily bread.

If the seed were to develop without interventions of any kind, if the seed were to evolve without interference of any sort, if sexual abuses did not exist, then upon becoming twenty-one years old, we would possess an extraordinarily energetic potential and we would conquer our little place under the Sun with great success.

It is good to know that many millions of inhabitants, many millions of people, are struggling to exist. There exist many millions of illiterate people who are suffering hunger and misery. One could protest against the government or governments and would solve nothing with such protests, because indeed, we should not blame others for our bad situation. We are the only ones responsible for our bad economic situation. We always blame the different political or economical systems, always accuse the president or presidents of the countries, and that is absurd, because we alone are the creators of our own destiny.

It is obvious that if we begin the struggle for life with weakness, if we do not possess the potent psychic-mental-erotic forces as to be able to carve our niche in life, we will suffer hunger and misery.

If the seed that one day entered the maternal womb had been allowed to harmoniously develop to the age of twenty-one, we would have entered the path of life with great success, strong and powerful, full of health and energy. Yet, unfortunately, most of us have been copulating since our second infancy, thus, we (as seeds that once entered the maternal womb) have not been able to successfully continue our process of development without hindrance.

As to the feminine sex, I will state that women develop earlier than men. Because of this, she can certainly marry at a younger age. Yet, for a teenager who is not yet a man, but a seed in the process of development, to marry before twenty-one years of age, to be copulating from the age of fourteen, is absurd, criminal and monstrous in the most complete sense of the word.

After the age of forty-two, that is to say, after the solar influence has elapsed during which we were to conquer our little place under the sun, we enter the age of Mars, which begins at the age of forty-two and lasts up to the age of forty-nine.

Whosoever ignores these cosmic cycles that repeat themselves in the human being, the microcosm, undoubtedly does not know how to take advantage of the cycle of Mars and he creates for himself a very miserable old age.

It is good that we think a little about old age, my dear friends; it is good that we begin preparing for old age. It is not right for us to wait until we are old to then try to arrange our existence.

Just as in our childhood we had a cradle, a home, a father, a mother, likewise in our old age we also need a house, we need a home. We need to have a source of financial income, enough so as not to perish of hunger and misery.

Between the ages of forty-two and forty-nine years old, the cycle of Mars is present, and in this period we should work very intensely to the maximum. It is during this time that we should give a concrete form to that home which we should have for our old age. It is between the age of forty-two and forty-nine years, under the influence of Mars, that we should create an economic source, which is absolutely secure for our old age.

Mars helps us with its energetic potential, but unfortunately, many have abused sex during the cycles of Venus and the Sun. When they arrive at the cycle of Mars, in spite of receiving the influence of this planet through their endocrine glands, they are totally worn out because of their sexual form of life, their abuses. Therefore, they in no way know how to take advantage, as they should, of their share of the potential. The result is lamentable, not taking advantage as they should of the cycle of Mars. Then, as a consequence or corollary, there arrives a miserable old age. Old age arrives and finds us without any secure source of income; and now, instead of being useful in some way or another, at least to our grandchildren, we undoubtedly become an obstacle for the entire world. All this, because of not knowing how to live! Because of not knowing how to live! Because of not knowing how to live!

From forty-nine to fifty-six years of age, thundering Jupiter enters our life, almighty Jupiter, he who gives the scepter to kings, the staff to patriarchs, and the horn of abundance to whomever deserves it.

However, if we have not really worked during the cycle of Mars, or if we have struggled at a disadvantage due to the abuse of sex, if we have not taken proper advantage of the solar influence and have not allowed the harmonious development of that seed that once entered that maternal womb, then the influence of Jupiter, instead of becoming positive, instead of granting us the scepter of kings, comes to give us misery.

Keep in mind that every planet has a dual aspect, positive and negative. If thundering Jupiter has as its ruler, the angel Zachariel, it also has as its dark antithesis, Sanagabril.

Distinguish between Zachariel and Sanagabril; they are different. Distinguish between the horn of abundance and the stick of the beggar. Obviously, whosoever has spent his sexual potential, has spent his vital values and his cosmic capital, reaps the consequences: misery, poverty, and humiliation in the cycle of Jupiter.

Old age, properly defined, begins at the age of fifty-six years with Saturn, the Ancient of the Heavens, and ends at sixty-three.

I do not necessarily mean that we must all die at the age of sixty-three. No, rather, that the first cycle of Saturn properly begins at fifty-six years and ends at sixty-three. Other cycles follow.

For example, the cycle of Uranus would then follow, but then only the internally developed individuals, the great Initiates, would grasp it.

The cycle of Neptune, with its seven years, would also be for the great Hierophants, followed by a cycle of Pluto for Mahatmas. Beyond that follow two transcendental cycles, and lastly, exquisite harmony and powers for those who have acquired the Elixir of Long Life.

In synthesis, the cycle of Saturn, for the human being of the streets, lasts seven years. On arriving at the age of sixty-three the cycle of Saturn ends.

For the common human being comes more combinations; for example: Saturn with the Moon or Saturn with Mercury. A similar change takes place every seven years, Saturn with Venus, etc.

That is why we see elderly people changing as the years go by. Take an old man or woman between sixty-three and seventy years old, for example, with Saturn and the Moon combining in him or her. They become very infantile in their way of being.

Between seventy and seventy-seven years, they would have a certain mercurial restlessness, certain desires to study or acquire knowledge, etc.

In any case, during old age, Saturn is combining in one form or another with the other worlds.

It is obvious that Saturn, the Ancient of the Heavens, is the sword of justice that reaches us from heaven. If we do not know how to live harmoniously with each of the planetary cycles, we will reap the results with Old Saturn, the Ancient of the Heavens.

Therefore, dear reader, these extraordinary, vital transformations of our own existence are marvelous. The ordinary human being thinks that on becoming twenty-one, one has come of age. Normally, yes; the seed that was born, or what one day entered the womb of existence and was then born alive to live, concludes its development at the age of twenty-one, that is precisely so.

Yet, if we were to fulfill our cosmic duty, as was done by our ancestors, the Lemurians and the Atlanteans, we would be converted into genuine Human Beings.

What is our cosmic duty? I will tell you of our cosmic duty:

FIRST: The **intellect**. Not to allow intellectual concepts to pass through our minds in a mechanical manner; in other words, I will state, become conscious of all the intellectual data that comes to the mind. How do we become conscious of this data? By means of

meditation. For example, when we read a book, we should meditate on it and try to comprehend it.

Second: The **emotions**. We should become conscious of all the activities of the emotional center. It is deplorable how people act under the impulse of emotions, in a completely mechanical manner, without any control whatsoever. We should become conscious of all our emotions.

Third: The habits and customs of the **motor center**. We should become conscious of all activities, of all movements, of all our habits. Do nothing mechanically.

Fourth: **Instincts**. We should take possession of all of our instincts and subdue them. We should comprehend them in depth.

Fifth: Transmute the **sexual energy**. By means of the Sahaja Maithuna, we will unceasingly transmute our sexual energies.

Thus, in fulfilling our cosmic duty, it is obvious that our life will develop harmoniously. The Superior Existential Bodies of our Being will be formed, built in us, and thus, we will be in harmony with the Infinite, attuned with the Great Law. We will be able to arrive at an old age full of ecstasy and conquer Mastery and Perfection.

Before the great Atlantean catastrophe that had completely changed the physiognomy of the terrestrial globe, and even before the abominable Kundabuffer organ of the continent of Mu had been developed, human beings fulfilled their cosmic duty and could then live, dear reader, a thousand years.

When one fulfills his cosmic duty, life prolongs itself. Unfortunately, the intellectual animal mistakenly called a human being became totally degenerated when he developed in his inner constitution the abominable Kundabuffer organ.

It is obvious that after having lost that organ, the consequences remained: the ego, the "I," the myself, within us. Once having these consequences, we became perverse, no longer wanting to carry out our cosmic duty and life became miserably shortened. In other times, when humanity was not yet degenerated, when it still fulfilled its cosmic duty, it was clear that existence could be prolonged. Any human being could reach an average of a thousand years of age. The results were that the Superior Existential Bodies of the Being were formed in each creature, and it was during this era that many Solar Men and Women, many Devas, many Divine Men appeared upon the face of the Earth.

Today one hardly sees these beings, because people do not fulfill their cosmic duty. It is therefore necessary to live attuned with the Infinite, to fulfill our cosmic duty, to become conscious of ourselves, and not to waste our sexual energies. We must teach our children to transmute the sperm into energy, warn them that it is a disgrace, a monstrosity to copulate before the age of twenty-one. Let adolescents know that they have not yet completed their process of development and that it is monstrous for a seed to be copulating. Seeds are seeds and they should develop.

Therefore, dear reader, meditate on all this, utilize Sexual Alchemy in yourselves so that you can accomplish these transmutations of the metallic planets within yourself.

It is through Sexual Alchemy, through the fulfilled cosmic duty, that we can transform old, aged Saturn into the Divine Moon, into that juvenile child.

It is by Sexual Alchemy, as I have already stated, that we can convert thundering Jupiter into the wise Mercury of secret philosophy.

It is through Alchemy that bellicose Mars can be transformed into a creature of love, and we can, thus, genuinely be born as Adepts.

The important thing is, I repeat, for our seed to develop harmoniously and that it then continues with the processes of ultra development until it achieves the Intimate Self-realization of our Inner Being.

Inverencial Peace.

Samael Aun Weor

Part I

Endocrinology

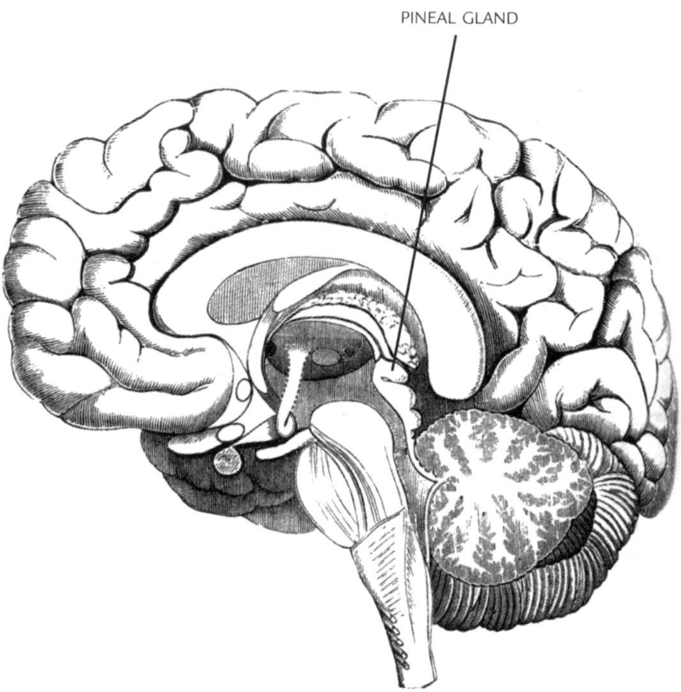
PINEAL GLAND

Chapter 1

The Pineal Gland

The pineal gland is situated in the posterior part of the brain. This small gland is only five millimeters in diameter. A very important, fine, sand-like tissue surrounds it. The pineal gland is a small tissue of a red-grayish color. This small gland is intimately related with the sexual organs. The pineal gland secretes certain hormones that regulate the whole process of evolution and the development of the sexual organs.

Conventional science assures that after these hormones have achieved their purpose, then this gland degenerates into a fibrous tissue. They state that after the total development of the sexual organs, the pineal gland is no longer capable of secreting any hormones.

Descartes assured us that this gland is the "seat of the Soul." The Orientals assure us that this gland is a dormant "third eye." When the occidental medicine of the world discovered that this gland is only a red-grayish tissue situated in the posterior part of the brain, then it rejected the affirmation of Descartes and the Orientals. It would have been better not to have created scientific dogmas and to have studied instead all the concepts in an eclectic and didactic form.

The yogis of India assure us that the pineal gland is the window of Brahma, the Diamond Eye, the polyvoyant eye, that through some special training, gives us the perception of the Ultra.

Occidental science should study these concepts of the oriental yoga. Occidental science is not the whole science. It is urgent also to study oriental science. We need a total, integral culture.

The microscope allows us to perceive objectively that which is infinitely small. The telescope allows us to see the infinitely grand. If the pineal gland allows us to see the Ultra of all things, then we should study the oriental yoga and develop that wonderful gland. The yogis of India have practices through which one can obtain a special superfunction of the pineal gland. Then we perceive the Ultra. To deny this affirmation of the oriental yoga is not scientific.

It is necessary to study and analyze.

The oriental sages say that sexual potency depends on the potency of the pineal gland. Now we can explain to ourselves the scientific basis of chastity.

There is no doubt that all the great Biblical prophets were great pinealists. Scientific chastity combined with certain practices permitted them to see the Ultra of Nature.

Gnostics state that the atom of the Holy Spirit is found within the pineal gland. Biology is resolved to investigate all these things. The Orientals affirmed that in the pineal gland is found the lotus flower of a thousand petals. There is no doubt that this is the crown of saints.

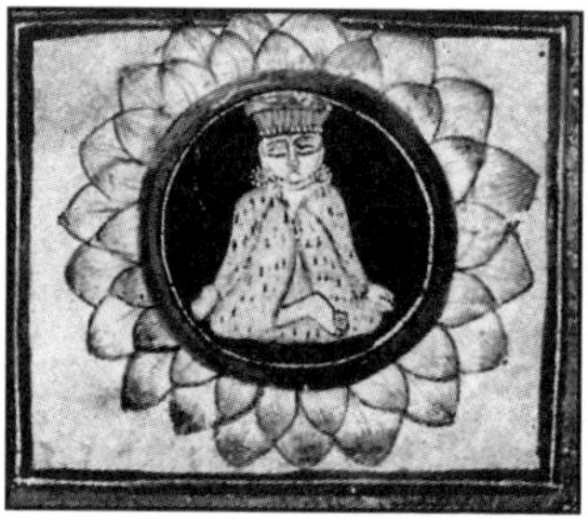
SAHASRARA CHAKRA

Human beings of great intelligence have their pineal gland highly developed. It has been discovered that the pineal glands of cretins are atrophied.

The great phenomena through which the masses become fascinated, so common in India, is only possible when the authentic Fakir has the pineal gland full of great vigor.

The blood directly absorbs the secretions of the endocrine glands. The blood bears all the secretions of the endocrine glands to other organs and glands that then are forced to be pushed in a major effort to a more intense work. The word *hormone* comes from a Greek word that means "to excite." Indeed, the hormones have the power of exciting the whole organism and obligate it to work.

The secretions of the endocrine glands also have influence over the mind. We now see why the Hindustani dedicate themselves to control the mind. Through our mind we can regulate our hormonal functions.

Some Hindustani sages have remained buried for many months without dying.

Biology cannot remain indifferent to all this. Biologists need to investigate all these wonders of Asia.

Mr. Emmanuel Kant admits a "nissus formativus" to our physical body. The oriental sages believe that the "nissus formativus" is a fluidic body that is found in contact with the Grand Sympathetic Nervous System and with the fluid nervous system. There is no doubt that this fluidic body is the Astral Body mentioned by medieval doctors. The human mind and all those purely psychic principles are within the Astral Body.

The senses of this Astral Body seem to bloom like lotus flowers from the very essence of the endocrine glands. The lotus of a thousand petals, mentioned by yogis of India, is a psychic sense of the Astral Body.

The special development of the pineal gland allows us to perceive the Astral Body and its psychic senses as lotus flowers bloom from the endocrine glands.

Medical science plays with the mechanism of phenomena, yet it does not know its vital depth. The special development of the pineal gland allows us to see the very vital depth.

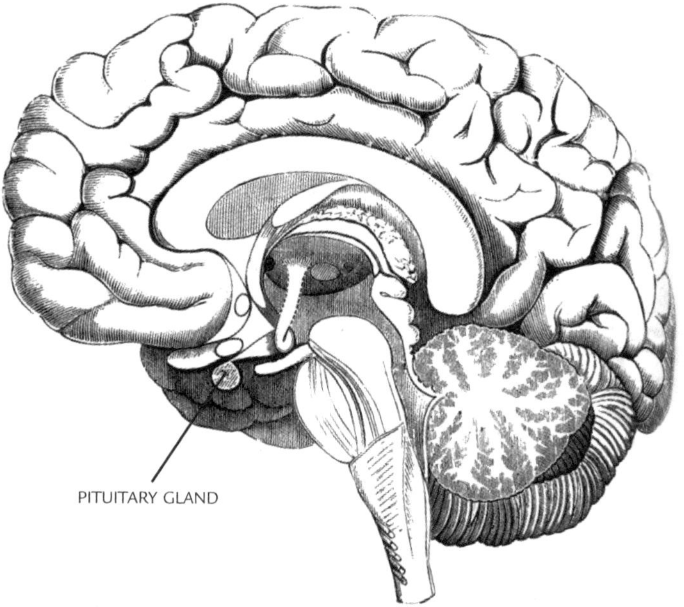
PITUITARY GLAND

Chapter 2

The Pituitary Gland

The pituitary gland is very small. Biology affirms that this gland is just the size of a pea and that it marvelously hangs from the very base of the brain and harmoniously rests over the sphenoid bone. We find a marvelous trinity related with this gland. The Law of the Triangle rules everything created.

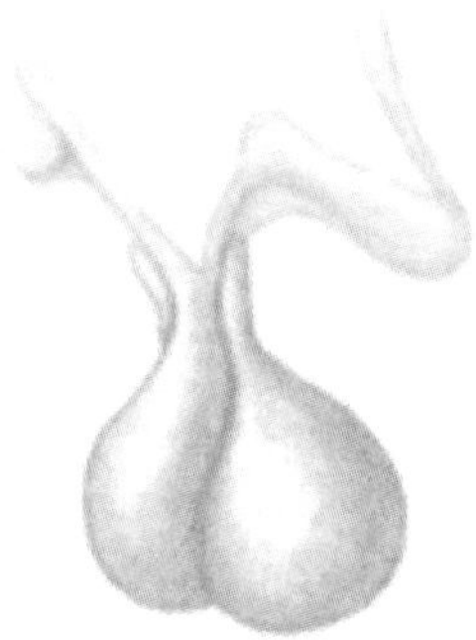

Indeed, three parts, two lobes and a middle, form the pituitary gland. Behold, here is the triangle, marvelous Law of All Creation. Biologists believe that life is absolutely impossible without the frontal or posterior lobe of the pituitary gland.

The frontal lobe of this gland is in charge of administering the size of the structure of the cellular community. Now then we must also know that within this administration there is also regulation and control. This is the only way we can explain to ourselves how life becomes impossible without the frontal lobes of the pituitary gland.

The hyperfunction of the frontal lobe of the pituitary originates gigantic human beings. When the function of the frontal lobes is insufficient then dwarves are the outcome. Therefore, it is logical to suppose that without the frontal lobe of the pituitary gland, life would be impossible, since this gland regulates the size of the structure of the cellular community.

Some forms of idiocy and blindness are also due to some abnormalities of the frontal lobe of the pituitary.

The function of the posterior lobe of the pituitary gland is to wonderfully invigorate the involuntary muscles of the organism. The secretion of the pituitary also effects the excretion of water from the kidneys.

Doctors use the pituitary to aid them in cases of difficult birth. Master H.P. Blavatsky stated that the pituitary gland is the page and light bearer of the pineal gland. Dr. Krumm-Heller, professor of medicine at the University of Berlin, stated that between the pituitary and pineal glands exists a small, very subtle channel or capillary. This channel or capillary is not found in dead bodies. Thus, these two glands are found connected by this fine channel.

There is no doubt whatsoever about electrobiology and the bioelectromagnetic forces. Why then, is a bioelectromagnetic interchange between the pineal and pituitary glands not accepted? The time has come to start analyzing all mystic sensorial and psychosomatic possibilities without fanaticisms, prejudices and dogmatisms.

The yogis of Hindustan state that the lotus of two petals sprouts from the pituitary gland. The occidental scientists, instead of laughing at these affirmations, should study them profoundly. To laugh at what we do not know is not scientific.

That lotus flower is found situated in the Astral Body exactly between the eyebrows. The sages of Hindustan give these lotus flowers the name of *chakras*. The yogis assure us that the pituitary chakra makes us clairvoyant. Many secret practices for the development of clairvoyance exist in the Holy Land of the Vedas. The Hindustani state that these chakras have eight major powers and thirty-six minor.

The clairvoyant can perceive the Ultra of nature. The clairvoyant can see the Astral Body. All the psychic and spiritual principles of the human being are found within the Astral Body. The clairvoyant perceives the fourth dimension.

Glandular energetics cannot be denied by biologists. The bioelectromagnetic interchange of the pineal and pituitary glands makes us clairvoyant.

There seems to exist a certain relationship between the atom of copper and the pituitary gland. Some sages utilize the element copper to develop clairvoyance. Nostradamus remained hours gazing at the waters contained inside a receptacle of pure copper. This wise physician (Nostradamus) made prophecies that have come true with exactitude throughout time. The astrologists assure us that Venus influences the pituitary gland and Venus also influences copper. Only this way can we comprehend the intimate relationship that exists between copper and the pituitary gland.

When the Catholic priests who arrived from Spain during the times of the Conquistadors came across a group of Aztec priests, something very interesting occurred. Traditions state that when the Catholic priests were catechizing some natives, they told them of angels and archangels, etc. After their talk, the autochthonous priests invited the Catholic priests to eat. The story goes that among the foods that the Catholic priests ate was a tasty cactus. This cactus momentarily gave clairvoyance to the Spanish priests. The Catholic priests then saw angels and archangels; so terrific was their amazement that they did not know what to do. Meanwhile, the autochthonous priests smiling said, "These angels and archangels of which you spoke, we already know them."

The account goes on to say that the Catholic priests had every one of the Aztec priests killed considering them wizards and magicians. There is no doubt about the power that these cactuses have for the instantaneous awakening of clairvoyance to those who eat it. This cactus is the peyote.* In the state of Mexico one cannot find peyote that is usable for clairvoyance. Whosoever wishes to find it must look for it either in Chihuahua or San Luis Potosi, Mexico. One must chew on it. The only good peyote is the ripe one. If it is dry, it is useless.

Biology cannot underestimate the peyote nor assure in a dogmatic and intransigent way that clairvoyant perceptions are hallucinations. Similarly, if the first sages who were able to see germs with the microscope were told and assured that such germs did not exist, that what they were seeing through the lens was nothing more than hallucinations, then in this day and age, we would still be ignoring the existence of germs.

Therefore, we need to be less dogmatic and more studious. We need to be more eclectic and more didactic.

The pituitary gland secretes seven types of hormones. The value of the pituitary gland in obstetrics is incalculable.

Dr. George Adoum, famous Gnostic writer and Grand Master of Higher Mysteries of the White Lodge, stated that the atom of the

---

* Editor's Note: Excerpted from *Aztec Christic Magic:* "We do not recommend the use of this marvelous cactus... Indeed, what we recommend is practice, much practice and soon you will act and travel within the astral body."

Cosmic Christ is found within the pituitary gland while the atom of the Father is found within the magnetic field at the root of the nose.

Biology analyzes and studies the scientific concepts of all sages. Biology came out from the horrible materialism of the eighteenth century, thus now it is starting to study all the physical, psychic and spiritual potencies of the internal secretions of the glands.

Chapter 3

The Thyroid Gland

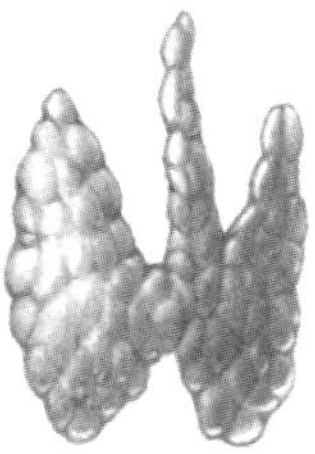

The Thyroid Gland

The thyroid gland is of a beautiful dark red color. The thyroid has two lobes that the endocrinologists know very well. The biologists amaze themselves looking at these two beautiful lobes wisely united by a wonderful isthmus. Behold here the perfect triangle.

The two lobes of the thyroid gland are found situated exactly at each side of the Adam's apple.

The thyroid gland is exposed to two fundamental sicknesses: Hyperthyroidism and Hypothyroidism. The first one is characterized by too much secretion, the second by too little secretion. Hyperthyroidism can be cured by surgery. Hypothyroidism cannot in any way be cured by surgery. Hypothyroidism is only possible to cure when the patient is given Thyroxine (a principle of secretion of the thyroid gland.) In reality, Thyroxine is an iodine compound very important in medicine.

Thyroxine is found intimately related with the whole metabolism of the physical body. When the patient suffers Hyperthyroidism, the excess of Thyroxine increases intensively the combustion of foods. The result is an increasing rhythm of normal respiration and heart rate.

In Hypothyroidism, the metabolism becomes slower. If a child were to suffer of Hypothyroidism, body and brain development would retard horribly. When Hypothyroidism is present in an adult, he becomes mentally weak. His nails and hair grow in a slow and abnormal form. Any physical strain fatigues him terribly and his skin becomes dry, flaky and somewhat bulky.

The biological iodine disinfects the whole organism. Without the biological iodine of the thyroid, our human organism would not be able to live. The Rosicrucian doctors assure us that Venus influences the thyroid gland and that Mars influences the parathyroid glands. The famous Dr. Arnold Krumm-Heller, professor of medicine at the University of Berlin, assures that between Venus and Mars there is a terrible struggle that repeats itself between the thyroid and parathyroid glands.

On a certain occasion, an old farmer who did not know how to read or write assured us that he had cured himself from the sickness of goiter by applying to himself a plaque of lead. The farmer told us that he made two small perforations with the purpose of tying a thread or cord. With that cord he tied the plaque around his neck, leaving the plaque over the root of the goiter. The farmer assured us that during the three months he wore the plaque, he was cured radically. He also mentioned to us that some family members also have cured themselves with the plaque of lead.

Metal Therapy is practically in an embryonic state. There is no doubt of the great possibilities of Metal Therapy. We have known some South American peasants that utilize salt and saliva, applying it during breakfast as the only remedy for the goiter. They mix these two elements during the waning of the moon and then apply it. This was their only remedy for the curing of such an ugly sickness. Biology is willing to study profoundly all these therapeutic systems of the peasants, because we are convinced that many of those formulas that our grandmothers used saved the lives of many illustrious personages.

The yogis of India state that the root of the laryngeal chakra comes out of the thyroid gland. The great doctor of the Hindustan Sivananda assures us that the laryngeal chakra has sixteen lotus petals.

Many occidental scientists laugh at what they do not know. The oriental sages state that a super-ear exists that is capable of registering the waves from the Ultra. They denominate that super-ear Clairaudience.

The laryngeal chakra is the center of Clairaudience. This demonstrates to us the intimate relationship between the thyroid gland and the mind.

If the thyroid gland and the mind are found so closely interrelated, why not admit the oriental theses on the chakra of the thyroid and its conceptual synthesis is valid?

The sages of India state that they achieve conceptual synthesis by developing the laryngeal chakra.

Physics accepts the Ether. The Hindustani state that Ether is but a condensation of the tattva Akasha. The great Asian yogis state that matter is the condensation of the Ether, and Ether, at the same time, is a condensation of the tattva Akasha, in which they find the ultimate synthesis, the primordial root of matter. The Hindustani consider the Akasha to be the primordial sound, and that its instrument in the human being is the creative larynx.

Doctor Sivananda assures us that with the development of the thyroid chakra, we can control Akasha, and we can achieve life during the profound night of the Great Pralaya.

According to Doctor Sivananda, eminent endocrinologist and Hindustani yogi, by awakening the chakra of the thyroid gland, we achieve Clairaudience. If one submerges into daily meditation with the purpose to hear a distant friend, then during the period of sleep one would be able to hear his words. With the interior meditation, one can awaken Clairaudience.

The secretions of the endocrine glands are found intimately related with all the order and control of the autonomous nervous system of the so-called involuntary muscles.

The glandular secretions govern, with great physiological-cosmic wisdom, the whole wonderful metabolism of the physical body. The endocrine secretions control the growth and development of all the grand cellular community.

The secretions of the endocrine glands control the characteristics of sexuality.

The thyroid gland has an auric radiation that is truly wonderful.

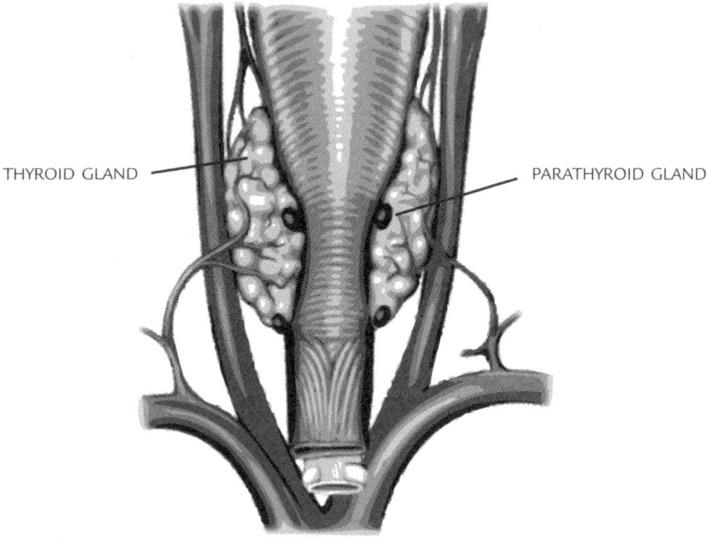
THYROID GLAND
PARATHYROID GLAND

Chapter 4

The Parathyroid Glands

The parathyroid glands should never be removed, because it has been proven that terrible convulsions and inevitable death can occur.

The two pairs of parathyroid glands normally regulate in a very amazing, knowledgeable way all the calcium values that are abundant in the cells and blood.

The secretions of the four wonderful parathyroid glands have to carry out the whole labor of calcium control in the cells and the blood.

This difficult job is possible thanks to the secretions of the four parathyroid glands.

Indeed, these glands are very small and are situated over each side of the thyroid.

Observing attentively, the biologists would be able to see a pair of small bodies the size of a pea.

Astrology sustains that Mars regulates these glands.

Conventional science only sees the glands from a very materialistic point of view.

The science of the Gnostic sages goes beyond.

In all atoms exist a triad of Matter, Energy, and Consciousness. Every cell is a triad composed of Matter, Energy and Consciousness.

Each gland of internal secretion is a truly microcosmic laboratory. The interrelation between the glands of secretion, the wise interchange of biochemical products, and the infinite perfection in which the glands work is showing us to satiation the existence of certain intelligent coordinates whose root we must search for in the Cosmic Consciousness.

Wherever there is life, there exists the consciousness. Consciousness is inherent to life as humidity is inherent to water. The yearning for consciousness and spirituality cannot be repressed.

In Soviet Russia there exist today fifteen million Muslims. It is evident that the materialism of Marx has failed totally.

Every machine is organized according to laws. Every machine has its rudder, its lever from which it is governed, and a pilot who controls it and conducts it. Why then should our human organism be an exception? The human body is a perfect machine built in the workshop of Nature by the Cosmic Consciousness. This machine has its rudder and lever from which it is governed and conducted.

That rudder is the Sympathetic Nervous System. The pilot that controls this machine is the Innermost (The Holy Spirit). Therefore, the Innermost wrapped in the Astral Body controls, by means of the Sympathetic Nervous System lever, the whole organism and all the hormonal secretions.

Chapter 5

The Thymus Gland

When the human being passes beyond sexual maturity, the thymus gland enters into decrepitude. This has already been proven.

The thymus gland is located at the very base of the neck.

The thymus gland has a very irregular form and structure.

This gland is intimately related to the mammary glands. Now we can explain to ourselves why the maternal milk is totally irreplaceable.

The thymus gland regulates the vitality of the child.

The astrologists say that the Moon influences this gland. The Gnostic sages want to conserve this gland and not let it fall into decrepitude.

When this gland is active, the organism does not age. The sage-doctors of antiquity said that the vowel "**A**," when it is pronounced wisely, has the power to make the thymus gland vibrate. The ancient sages utilize the wise mantra so vulgarized by people today: **Abracadabra**. This mantra is said to keep the thymus gland active during life. They pronounced this word forty-nine times in the following way:

Abracadabra
Abracadabr
Abracadab
Abracada
Abracad
Abraca
Abrac
Abra
Abr
Ab
A

The word was pronounced so that the sound of the vowel "**A**" was prolonged. Even some doctors are beginning to cure by means of musical sound. It is interesting to acknowledge that in the voice of the doctor, in each of his words, there is a source of life or death to his patients.

The endocrinological science should study the intimate relationships that exist between music and the endocrine glands. It is better to investigate, analyze, and comprehend than to laugh at that which we do not know.

When a child is hungry, the mother must breast feed him. The books on maternity that recommend a child go hungry for so many hours are a crime against public health.

This matter of the human being wanting to correct nature is manifestly absurd. When the infant cries in hunger, it is a crime against nature to deny him food.

Chapter 6

The Heart

The heart is truly a double pump. One side of the heart pumps blood in one direction while the other pumps blood in the opposite direction. These two pumping directions complement and harmonize each other wonderfully. The most interesting thing about the two opposite blood streams pumped by the heart is that they do not collide but help each other to mutually advance.

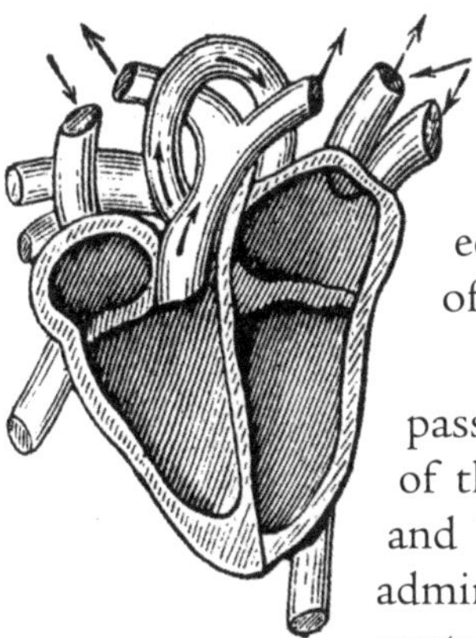

The heart is truly the Sun of our organism. The heart is the greatest wonder of creation. Nevertheless, there exist persons eminently cultured and educated who do not know the physiology of the heart.

It is something to admire, to see the passage of blood through that swift river of the aorta. This artery is truly a mighty and beautiful river. We fill ourselves with admiration and mystical beauty when contemplating that grand river full of life. This grand river ramifies into minor rivers, small arteries and then into small creeks that carry life to all parts, to nourish and give life to millions of small micro-organisms (cells, genes, etc.) All those organisms are a triad of matter, energy, and consciousness. All those beings of the infinitely small adore us like a God. The smallest creeks of the blood are the capillary vessels. The cells of the diverse tissues and organs are found inside the weft of the capillary networks.

Thus, the cells live from the blood streams pumped by the heart. The cells are composed of molecules and atoms. Each atom is a true universe in miniature. Every atom is a triad of matter, energy, and consciousness. The Nous Atom, which lives in the left ventricle of the heart, governs the atomic intelligences.

The suction atoms of the heart obey orders of the Nous Atom and transmit them to the engineer atoms that conduct the activity

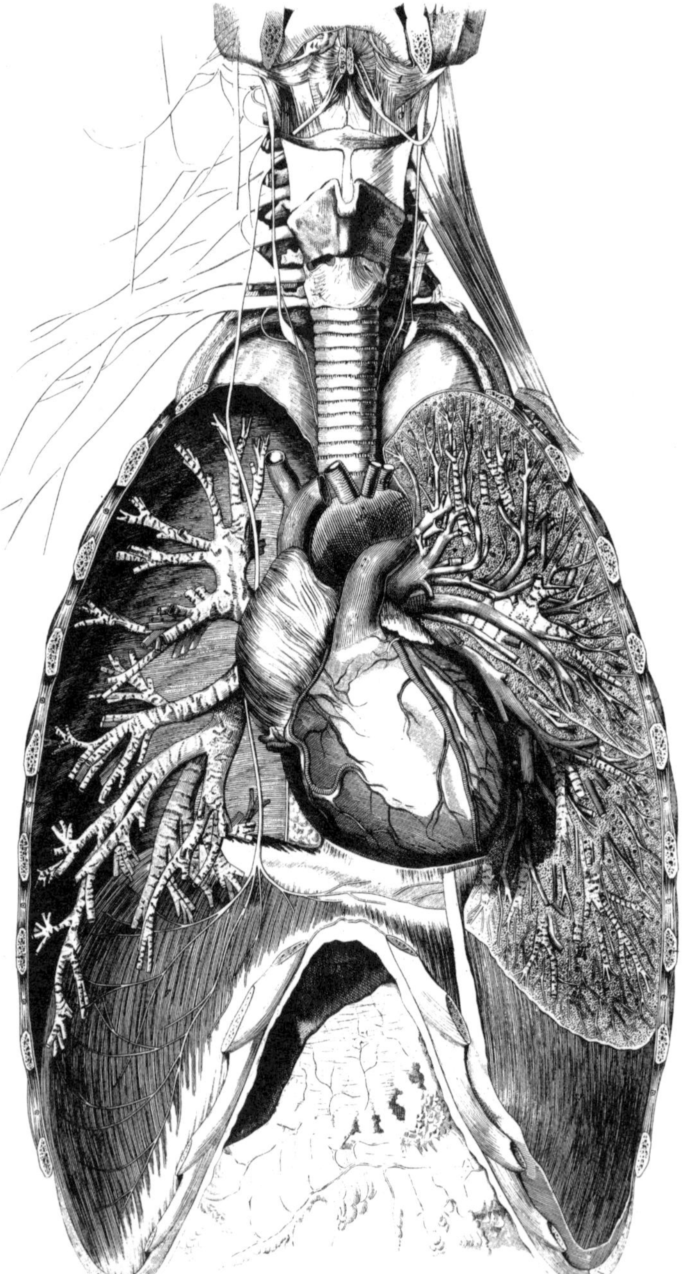

The Heart and the Lungs

of each organ. The atomic workers of each organ obey orders from the engineer atoms and work according to those orders.

There also exist a multitude of indolent atoms that cause diseases. The Nous Atom of the heart works under the direction of the Architect Atom and the latter under the orders of the Innermost.

The heart is a shallow muscle about the size of the fist, that looks more or less like a pear. The heart contracts, expands, and relaxes incessantly. This is the ebb and tide of the grand Ocean of Life. Every life has its systole and diastole. Everything pulses and repulses in the infinitely small, as well as in the infinitely grand. "As above, so below." This is the law of the grand life.

In the heart exist two wonderful polarities: positive and negative. These are like two hearts incessantly pumping blood into two opposite directions. The two compartments of the heart have two chambers, a superior and an inferior. The superior chambers are the auricles. The inferior chambers are the ventricles. The Secret Doctrine recognizes Seven Secret Chambers in the heart and Seven Secret Cavities in the brain.

There exist a right auricle and a right ventricle. There exist a left auricle and a left ventricle. The superior chambers from right to left are the auricles. The inferior chambers from right to left are the ventricles.

Meditating on the heart lotus, we control the tattva Vayu (Air Principle), and the power over winds and hurricanes is granted. The Hindustani state that the lotus flower of the heart has fifteen wonderful petals. The whole intimate functionalism of the heart, its whole vital profoundness must be searched in the lotus flower of fifteen petals whose subtle stem emanates from the Heart Temple.

The vena cava, full of organic wastes, deposits blood into the heart. The right auricle receives the impure bloodstream and wisely passes it to the right ventricle that is beneath. A few instants later, the right ventricle pumps its blood charged with lymph and wastes through its valve to pass it to the interior of the lung by means of the pulmonary artery.

The Cosmic Intelligences have not neglected anything. It is interesting for the sage to contemplate this whole functionalism.

It is wonderful to see the Great Pulmonary Artery divide itself into the two smaller arteries, one for each lung.

Inside the lungs, the pulmonary arteries ramify also, until they become minute capillary vessels. Each drop of blood has to pass inevitably through the capillary vessels of the lungs, where it delivers the excess anhydrous carbon and absorbs, in exchange, the exceeding oxygen.

The rich oxygenated blood penetrates intelligently into the small veins and then to the larger veins. The two great pulmonary arteries deposit their rich blood charged with oxygen into the left auricle of the heart. The blood has exchanged its excess of anhydrous carbon for oxygen. Now with life renewed from the left auricle, the blood passes to the left ventricle and then through the aorta under the rhythmic impulse of the heart and follows at last into all the arteries and sangineous vessels. In all this work we can see the intimate relationship that exists between Vayu (Air Principle) and the heart.

Therefore, the Hindustani are not too far off when they associate Vayu (Air Principle) with the heart. This demonstrates to us the physiological-cosmic knowledge that the Orientals possess concerning the heart organ.

Why do the occidentals not want to study the oriental Yoga? Why do the occidentals want to laugh at what they do not know? It would be wiser to study Sivananda, the great yogi. (The book entitled *Kundalini Yoga* is a prodigy of oriental wisdom.)

Those who wish to put their body in a Jinn state, those who want to learn to put their physical body in the fourth dimension, must develop the lotus of the heart. A yogi with his body in a Jinn state can fly through the air, walk on water, as did Jesus Christ on the Sea of Galilee, or walk through fire without burning as many yogis of India do. A yogi with his body in a Jinn state can go through rocks as the disciples of Buddha did.

The lotus of the heart develops with meditation and prayer. The occidental doctors say that the heart produces two sounds, one low pitched and muted and the other loud and high pitched, "lub" and "dub." The physiologists assure us that the first sound is pronounced immediately after the contraction of the ventricles, and that the second is due to the closing of the valves that separate the ventricles of the aorta and the pulmonary artery. The Hindustani doctors go further because they have refined their senses. The yogis of India state that in the heart there exist ten mystic sounds.

The first sound is like the voice of the Son of Man.

The second is the sound of the chibini.

The third is the sound of the great cosmic bell.

The fourth is the internal thundering of the Earth.

The fifth is the delightful sound of the laud.

The sixth is the cymbal of the Gods.

The seventh is of the enchanted flute.

The eighth is of the big drum.

The ninth is of the double tambi.

The tenth is the sound of the seven thunders that in the apocalypse repeat the voices of the Eternal One.

If the sounds heard by the Occidental doctors are true, why can not the ten sounds of the Oriental be true?

If the two sounds of the Occidental doctors have been demonstrated, why should not the ten Oriental sounds be demonstrated?

Everything is a question of demonstrative scientific procedures. The Occidentals have their demonstrative scientific procedures. The Orientals also have their demonstrative scientific procedures.

The Oriental concentrates mentally and meditates on the ten mystic sounds. The Oriental mind absorbs itself in the ten mystic sounds. Hence, the yogi's "Nissus Formativus" or the Astral Body of the medieval doctors (within which there are all the psychic and spiritual principles of the human being), leaves the physical body in ecstasy within the ten mystic sounds of the heart. This is the Samadhi of the Hindustani Yogis. Thus, this is how the yogi transports himself to the most distant worlds of the Infinite.

Instead of laughing and criticizing these matters that they have neither studied nor experimented, the occidental scientists should study the yoga.

The Hindustani state that inside the chakra of the heart exists a hexagonal space of an ineffable black color. There exist the ten mystic sounds.

Occidental minds laugh at all these. If the occidental scientists would develop clairvoyance they would see and stop laughing.

Doctors are able to photograph the heartbeat. This is done with the instrument called the electrocardiograph. It is wonderful to see how they totally synchronize all the heartbeats, all the chambers, as if there were only two. This is only possible thanks to that handful of nerves. This handful of nerves, also called the ventricular atrium, automatically synchronize in a wonderful form the two auricles in a single weak heartbeat contraction, and the two ventricles in a single strong heartbeat contraction.

If the electrocardiograph is capable of photographing the heartbeats, how much more would he who develops clairvoyance see? A new world opens before the clairvoyant, an infinite world of immeasurable variety.

Within the heart is the Internal Christ of any human being who comes to the world. He is our real Being.

Chapter 7

The Pancreatic Gland

The pancreas happens to be a gland partially without a tube. All the digestive juices of the human organism empty into the duodenum through the famous tube of Wirsung.

The famous Dr. Arnold Krumm-Heller, professor of medicine at the University of Berlin, stated in his *Zodiacal Course* that the constellation of Virgo has influence over the womb and especially over the barren islet of Langerhans.

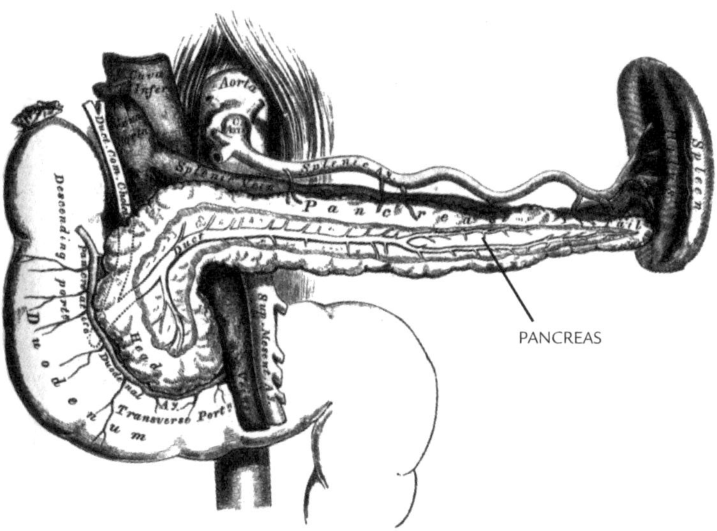

Insulin is important because it governs all the metabolism of the carbohydrates. The barren islets of the pancreas secrete insulin.

When the barren islets of the pancreas do not function properly, diabetes develops. The principal work of the barren islets is to secrete insulin correctly, and the principal work of the pancreas is the transformation of sugars. When the sugars go directly to the blood steam, this is diabetes.

With the treatments of insulin, medical science has achieved control of diabetes. However, it has not cured diabetes. We have known many diabetic patients that have been cured with the famous antibiotic tea. The formula of this tea is as follows:

- 30 grams of avocado leaves
- 30 grams of eucalyptus tree leaves
- 30 grams of walnut tree leaves

Boil the three ingredients in a liter of water.

Dose 3 glasses daily, one before each meal.

Drink for six consecutive months.

This harmless tea has no adverse effect on the insulin treatment.

The secretion of the islets of Langerhans passes directly to the blood. The Hindustani state that above the navel is found the lotus of ten petals. This chakra, situated in the region of the navel, controls the liver, stomach and the pancreas. The yogis state that the color of this chakra is like the clouds charged with lightning sparks and living fire.

The yogis of Hindustan that have developed this chakra of the navel can remain in the fire without burning. The sages of Hindustan state that within the chakra of the navel sparkles the Tejas tattva (Igneous Ether).

The occidental biologists state that this is impossible. The occidental sages should travel to Hindustan and investigate this. Many skeptical occidentals that have traveled to India came back amazed to see these yogis remain in the fire without burning.

The Hindustani yogis develop this chakra of the navel with concentration and meditation. They concentrate full hours on the navel. When certain occidental hypnotists traveled through those lands of Hindustan, Pakistan, the Great Tartary, Mongolia, China and Tibet and witnessed these oriental sects and saw this meditation on the navel, they believed it to be self-hypnosis. Actually it is quite the opposite. In truth, they put themselves through all these meditations and concentrations for hours in order to develop this chakra around the region of the navel.

Chapter 8

The Liver

The liver is the biggest gland of the organism. The liver is situated on the right side, exactly below the diaphragm. The liver has a dark red color. The liver weighs four pounds, more or less, and is a little less than nine inches long, seven inches wide, and four inches across through its thickest part.

Doctors call the liver "the organ of the five." The Kabbalists know that the five is the number of Geburah, rigor, the Law. Many mystics state that Christ is crucified in the liver. There is no doubt that the liver is the seat of appetites and desires. From that point of view, we can really state that we have Christ crucified in the liver.

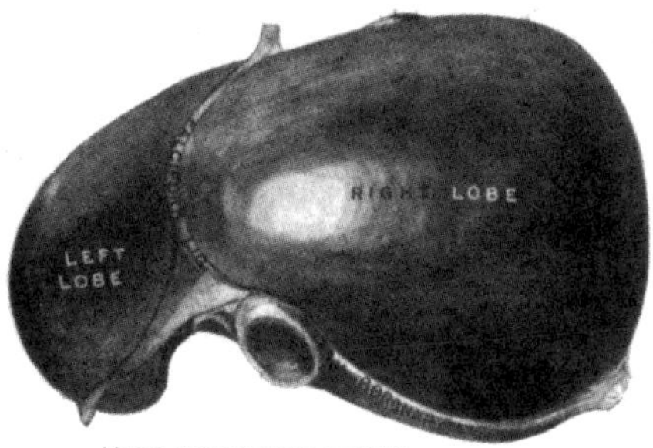

UPPER SURFACE VIEW OF LIVER

The liver possesses five admirable lobes, five groups of wise harmonic tubes, five wonderful sangineous vessels, and five basic functions.

The number five of the liver reminds us of the Law, the Nemesis that weighs on all those actions that are the offspring of desire and of all evil.

In the Liver of Brass, found in the ruins of Piacenza, were found the engravings of the twelve zodiacal signs. This invites us to think on the five of the liver. It is said that the ancient astrologists prognosticated by consulting the liver. They looked at the liver and forecasted.

The whole zodiac of the microcosmic human being has its own laws and its signs written in the liver.

The lobe of the liver comes to give unity to the whole structure of the liver. The lobe of the liver gives unity to the hepatic functions. When biologists study the hepatic gland, they are able to prove that the wonderful lobe of the liver comes to be something like a small liver in miniature. This is admirable! Whosoever totally comes to know the whole lobe of the liver knows practically the whole liver. The lobe of the liver is a mass of admirable cells united by a wonderful adjoining tissue. Each lobe contains five of six beautiful and perfect sides; each lobe possesses its own set of minute and beautiful vessels, its own secreting cells and its own tubes. A group of small hepatic lobes of the liver construct the liver itself. This is the Law of Five.

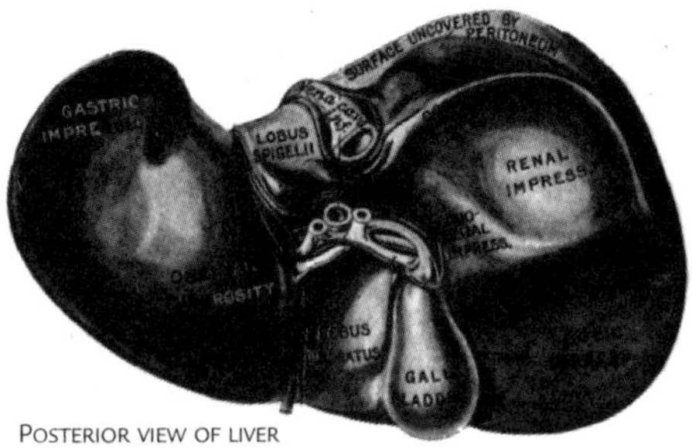

POSTERIOR VIEW OF LIVER

The cells of the liver secrete the bile so indispensable for the digestion of fats. The liver produces glucose so important for the tissues. This work of the transformation of sugar into glucose is an admirable work of Alchemy.

Certain internal secretions of the liver exist that regulate the alchemical transmutation of glucose and of glycogen into sugar.

The liver controls the calories of the organism. In its alchemical laboratory, the liver produces the substance called coagulase. The coagulase is an indispensable substance for coagulation.

All five functions of the liver are fundamental for the life of the organism. The liver is in charge of burning, in its alchemical laboratory, all the wasted and old cells, forming residues that are easily eliminated.

The hepatic artery gives the liver all the blood it needs. The adjoining tissue that enfolds the liver reaches to penetrate inside the organ itself and separate it into its five perfect divisions. Each small lobe of the liver is like an island surrounded by a multitude of sanguineous vessels.

The portal vein carries venous blood to the liver. This vein inside the liver ramifies into a multitude of vessels. Each small lobe of the liver has its own vein. Each cell of the small lobes of the liver is placed in a net of minute sanguineous vessels.

There also exist small interlobular veins. Each cell of the small lobes of the liver receives the venous blood proceeding from the stomach, spleen, pancreas and intestines through the famous portal vein that, like a river of pure life, takes nourishment to the liver. The barren islets of the cells of the liver receive their sanguineous nourishment from the small interlobular veins. Nothing is left without life in the liver. Everything receives life. Each cell of the liver is a true alchemical laboratory in charge of wisely transmuting the food into valuable substances for all the cells of the organism. All the transformed blood leaves through the small interlobular veins to pass to the interior of a vessel named the central vein.

The central vein drains off into that great abundant river known as the vena cava. The hepatic cells that live inside the liver like small conscious and intelligent workers have to transform many substances in the bile to help digestion. The bile remains in the bile duct until it is needed, then it is emptied into the duodenum.

The sages of Hindustan see clairvoyantly that from the hepatic gland emerges a lotus flower, the Hepatic Chakra.

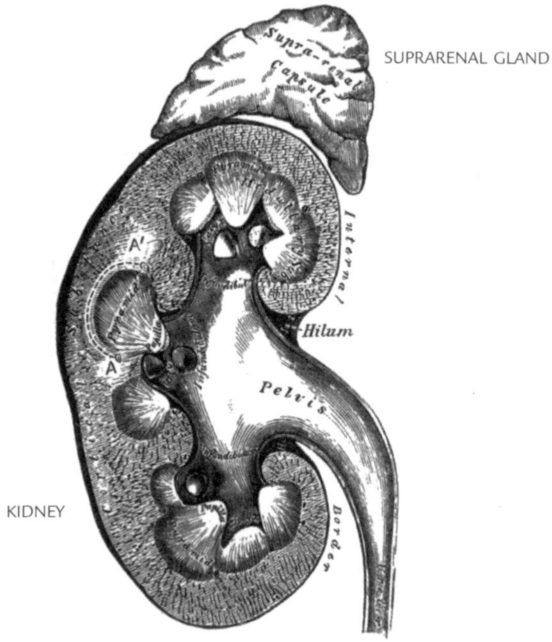

SUPRARENAL GLAND
KIDNEY
Supra-renal Capsule
Internal
Hilum
Pelvis
Border
A'
A

Chapter 9

The Suprarenal (Adrenal) Glands

Adrenaline (Epinephrine) is a very important hormone in the human organism. It serves to maintain the tone of the sanguineous vessel walls. The cortex of the suprarenal is intimately related with the development of the sexual glands. There exists no doubt about the influence so marked by the suprarenal cortex in relation to sex. The suprarenal cortex influences the development of the glands and above all the characteristics of sexuality. The famous doctor of medicine Paracelsus stated in regards to the kidneys the following:

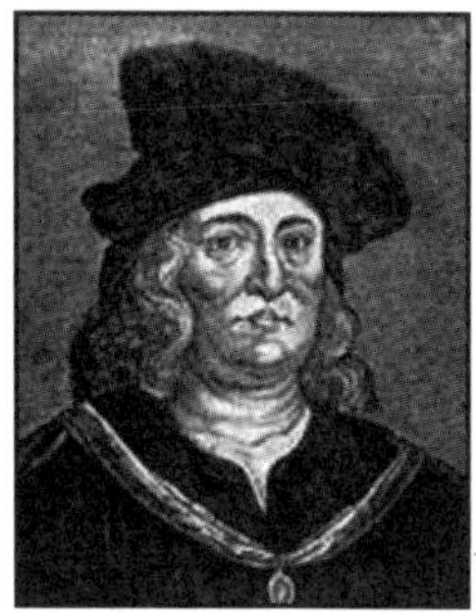
PARACELSUS

> "The nature and the exaltation of Venus is found in the kidneys in the grade and predestination that correspond to the planet or the entrails. Well then, since the operation that Venus performs is directed toward the fruits of the Earth that must be engendered, the potency of the kidneys concentrates itself on the human fruit."

Undoubtedly, Paracelsus was referring to the sexual organs with which Venus will never be able to exhaust the body. He continues:

> "It is natural that the kidneys perform this function, and indeed, no other organ could accomplish it better. Thus, when Venus, for example, receives the Great Entity, the potency of the conception, the kidneys dry their power of sentiment (Sensus) and of the will of man."

The doctors of psychoanalysis can prove the former statement that Paracelsus affirmed. The psychoanalysis of Freud has produced a true innovation in the field of medicine. The croakers who have not wanted to accept the psychoanalysis are retarded and antiquated.

The Yogis see two chakras in the kidneys, one on each kidney. The sages of Hindustan state that the chastity or fornication of a human being is marked in these two chakras. This brings to our attention that phrase in the Apocalypse of St. John that states:

> *I am he who searcheth the kidneys* (reins) *and hearts: and I will give unto every one of you according to your works.*
>
> - Revelation 2:23

The great clairvoyants see two lotus flowers, one on each kidney. They state that when the human being is a fornicator these flowers are of a bloody red color, and when he is chaste, they are of a white color.

The adrenal glands are situated in the superior part of the kidneys. These small yellow glands resemble true pyramids. Each adrenal gland has its own cortex and medulla that differ from each other in their structure and function.

The hormone of the adrenal cortex controls the sodium and potassium of the blood and the cells.

Psychoanalysis has demonstrated that in those instances of fear, pain, anger, etc, the adrenal medulla secretes a larger quantity of adrenaline that prepares all the cells of the organism to encounter all kinds of emergencies.

The dog is an animal that has a very fine sense of smell. When someone is afraid of him, the dog perceives the smell of adrenaline from the adrenal glands of the frightened person, and the dog may try to bite the person. The dog, by his sense of smell, knows who is afraid of him.

Excess adrenaline interferes negatively in digestion. Very strong emotions can cause indigestion.

Chapter 10

The Spleen

The spleen is a very important organ in the human organism. When the hour of sleep arrives, the soul, wrapped in the Astral Body, abandons the physical body and travels about the world of the fifth dimension. Meanwhile, something remains inside the physical body. This something is the Ethereal Double. The double is the Lingam Sarira of the sages of Hindustan. Dr. Paracelsus named that Ethereal Double the *Mumia*.

This Mumia is a double organism of ethereal matter. This Mumia is the vital seat, the vital depth of the physical body, which is absolutely unknown to occidental medicine. Yet it is known totally by oriental doctors.

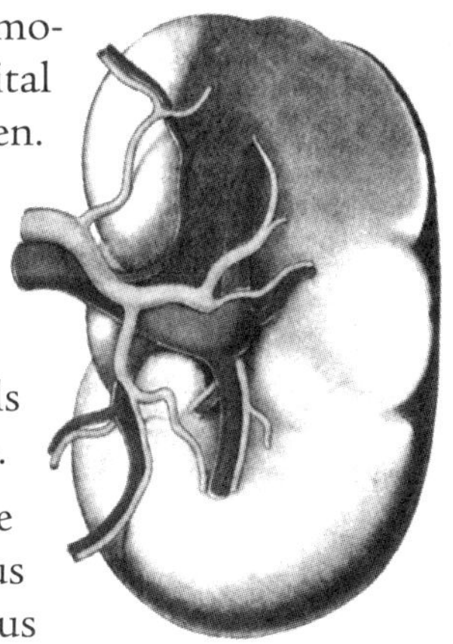

The Mumia of Paracelsus is a Thermo-electromagnetic condensation. The Vital Body has a fundamental chakra in the spleen. The lotus flower of the spleen specializes the vital currents of the Sun. The lotus flower of the spleen attracts the solar vital currents and absorbs them. We see then in the spleen that the white blood cells transmute themselves into red blood cells.

The vital energy collected by the Spleenic Chakra passes to the solar plexus and then spreads throughout all the nervous channels of the Grand Sympathetic system, filling the whole human organism with life.

The thyroid gland collaborates in this job with its biological iodine, disinfecting all the channels of the Grand Sympathetic Nervous System.

When the soul, wrapped in its Astral Body, reenters the physical body, the body is already repaired. If the conscious being were not to leave the physical body, then his emotions and thoughts would interfere with the reconstruction of his human organism.

During the day, many organic refuses are being accumulated in the canals of the Grand Sympathetic Nervous System. These organic refuse impedes the circulation of the vital fluid. Slumber is the outcome of this interference. Thus, during the sleep process, the human organism is reconstructed.

A medium in a trance state can project the Mumia through the spleen. This Mumia is then utilized by some disincarnated entities who enter within it. Afterwards, these entities physically condense or materialize. This is how it has been possible to have seen and touched some people that have been dead. This is not a fantasy because photographs have been taken of those persons that are already dead. The photographic plates cannot lie. Facts are facts.

The famous Dr. Louis Zea Uribe, professor of medicine in the National University of Bogota, was an atheist, materialist and skeptic one hundred percent. When this man saw, touched, and felt those phantoms that materialized in a laboratory in Naples, he then was transformed radically and became a spiritualist one hundred percent.

In a scientific laboratory in Naples the materializations that were made through the famous medium Eusapia Paladino were studied. Thus, the skeptic scientists saw, heard, photographed, experimented, and believed.

Chapter 11

The Vital Depth

The scientists that place doubt in the existence of Ether have no scientific basis for their theories. Indeed, they just play with words, with terms, because instead of the term Ether they use the term "radioactivity" or a "magnetic field," etc. So, these other terms neither take away from nor give to the reality of Ether. In any case, their doubts, analysis, and change of terms will only serve them to study that which is called Ether. Most of the time, people fight only for the question of terms of words, etc., etc. Yet, in the final analysis, what counts are the facts, and the facts are facts.

Russian astronomers have discovered, with their powerful telescopes, worlds in a protoplasmic state. These protoplasmic worlds have come out from within the Ether. We can accept, by simple logical induction, that Ethereal worlds exist. Maybe some scientists will not be pleased with the term "Ethereal." However, the term is of the least importance. The importance is the fact.

Every world, before becoming protoplasmic, exists in an Ethereal state. The great Hindustani scientist Rama Prasad stated: "Everything comes out from within the Ether. Everything returns into the Ether."

If protoplasm emerges from within the Ether, then we have to accept that the Ether is in the vital depth of everything that exists.

The oriental mystics consider that the Ethereal Body (vital depth) of the human body has four classes of Ether. This does not appeal to the occidental scientists. Nevertheless, when the occidental scientists study the Ether, no matter what name they will give to it, they then will have to accept by simple analysis and by their own experience, the reality of the four Ethers of the oriental mystics.

Thus, the Ethereal Body of a human being has four Ethers: Chemical Ether, Ether of Life, Luminous Ether, and Reflecting Ether. Each one of these Ethers has its function in intimate relation with the whole organic economy.

The **Chemical Ether** is related with all the processes of organic assimilation and nourishment.

The **Ether of Life** is related with the reproduction processes of the race.

The **Luminous Ether** is related with the processes of sensorial perception.

The **Reflecting Ether** is intimately related with the faculties of memory, imagination, willpower, etc., etc.

The Vital Body controls the whole motor vessel nervous system and is the seat of life. Each Ethereal atom penetrates inside each physical atom and makes it vibrate. If we definitely extract the Vital Body from the physical body of a person, this person dies inevitably. It is totally absurd to suppose, even for a moment, that chemical-physical organisms can survive without the Vital Body. The very atheist, materialist Russians, after having studied the matter profoundly, have become more prudent in giving consent about the Vital Depth of the living matter.

The scientists who are exploring the human organism are getting closer to the Ethereal Body. They will detect it inevitably and soon they will be able to condense it with some kind of ectoplasm to study it in a laboratory.

All the functions of our organism, all the caloric activities, the reproduction, combustion, metabolism, etc., have their base in the vital depth.

When the Vital Body weakens, then the diseases of the physical body appear.

Chapter 12

The Tattvas and Hormones

The Ether exists in an igneous state (Tejas). The Ether exists in a gaseous fluidic state as the origin of air (Vayu). The Ether exists in an aqueous state as the origin of water (Apas). The Ether exists in a petreous state as the origin of minerals (Prithvi).

These are the Tattvas of the Hindustani. When the Tattvas Tejas, Vayu, Apas and Prithvi materialize or condense, we have then the four physical elements, namely: Fire, Air, Water, and Earth.

Our Ethereal Body is formed by the Tattvas. The Tattvas and the chakras are intimately related. The Tattvas enter the Chakras and then pass into the interior of the glands of internal secretion. When the Tattvas are inside these minute endocrine laboratories (the glands), they intensify the glands' work by transforming themselves into hormones. Thus, the Tattvas enter the organism but do not leave it.

The Tattvas also transform themselves into genes and chromosomes that later on transform themselves into spermatozoids.

Everything comes from Ether. Everything returns into Ether.

The Ether is the condensation of a substance called Akasha. This substance, Akasha, is the first radiation of Mulaprakriti, which is its root or insipid and undifferentiated primordial matter. This Mulaprakriti is known among the Alchemists as the Ens Seminis, the entity of semen.

Akasha is therefore the igneous radiation of the primordial matter. Akasha is contained within the semen. The Alchemists state that water (semen) is the habitat of fire (Akasha). Akasha is therefore the Kundalini of the Hindustani.

In the books of genesis (from all religious literature), the primordial matter (Mulaprakriti) is represented by the waters. In the beginning, the protoplasm of any nebula is ethereal.

If we look further, we have to accept that behind each effect there exists a cause. Therefore, the Ether itself has to have a cause. We have learned from the yogis of Hindustan that the cause of

Ether is Akasha. The oriental sages state that Akasha is a sea of fire. This Super-astral Fire is contained within the Ens Seminis (the Mulaprakriti of the sages of India). The seed atoms of any known matter are the Ens Seminis. Akasha is Super-astral Fire. The sounds condense through the mediation of Akasha. The Kundalini serpent is fire and sound. Therefore, no one could incarnate the Word (Christ) without previously raising the sacred serpent, because it is impossible to concrete and materialize the sound without Akasha.

The Pranas Vayus are sounding waves of Akasha. These sounding waves condense themselves in the Tattvas of the Ether. The Tattvas materialize themselves in the four elements of Nature: Fire, Air, Water, and Earth. In conclusion, the chemical-physical world is the outcome of the materialization of sound. The chemical-physical world is condensed sound. We do not accept an anthropomorphic and dogmatic God, but scientifically, we accept sound as a *causa causorum* of the Universe.

Furthermore, a cause for the precosmic sounds has to exist. The great oriental sages tell us of a Solar Logos. Dr. Krumm-Heller stated that "the Logos sounds." Indeed, the Logos is the Word.

> *In the beginning was the Word, and the Word was with God and the Word was God. The same was in the beginning with God. All things were made by him; and without Him was not anything made that was made. In Him was life and the life was the light of men. And the light shineth in darkness; and the darkness comprehend it not.*
>
> JOHN 1:1-5

The Logos is not an individual. The Logos is an army of ineffable beings.

Chapter 13

The Prostate

This very important gland, the prostrate, is very small. Every man and male of the mammal species has one.

Examining very carefully, we can see that this wonderful gland is situated exactly at the neck of the bladder.

Modern science still does not totally know all the functions of the prostate.

The prostate secretes a white and viscous liquid.

The sages of medicine know that in women, the urethra measures only 35 millimeters and it is very dilatable. In man, it has been proven to be 20 to 27 centimeters in length.

The wizard-doctors from Egypt, Greece, Samothrace, Troy, India, etc., always gave a lot of importance to the prostate. Swami Sivananda, great yogi doctor of India, states that the lotus of the prostate has six petals.

Many beings live in the Ultra of Nature, in the fourth dimension, with their Solar Astral Bodies. The oriental sages state that they have cognizance of those beings thanks to their prostatic chakra. These great sages of Hindustan concentrate daily on their prostatic chakra. They imagine that their chakra rotates from left to right like a magnetic wheel, while vocalizing the letter "**M**" with the lips closed. The letter "**M**" sounds as if imitating the bellowing of a bull, but without that deepness of voice. This is a profound and vibrating sound. This practice will awaken the prostatic chakra if it is practiced daily through many years.

When the prostatic chakra enters into activity, it grants us the power to leave the physical body, to move in the Astral Body. This is how we are able to move in the Astral Body independent of physical matter. In the Astral Body, the human being can investigate for himself the great mysteries of life and death. The prostatic chakra grants us the power of astrally projecting the personality. The peyote is a Mexican cactus that produces the projection of the human personality. With the peyote, any human being can project himself in the Astral Body consciously.

This cactus plant does not have thorns but flowers of a whitish, pink color and its fruits of a light pink color. The ancient Aztecs worshipped the peyote as a sacred plant. The epidermis of this cactus is very smooth and it has from five to twelve sides that separate among themselves by beautiful lines of fine hairs.

The technical name of peyote is *Anhalonium Williamsil.* The peyote that is useful for the projection of the personality is not found in the Capital of Mexico nor in the whole state of Mexico. Whosoever wants to find legitimate peyote would have to look for it in Chihuahua among the Taumara Indians or in San Luis Potosi in Northern Mexico.

The plant must be chewed. This plant must be ripe and fresh. It is useless if it is dried. In the moment of chewing the cactus, the disciple must be concentrated on his Innermost, that is to say, on his own Internal Being. One must, in this moment, assume a mystical attitude. Let us remember that our Internal Being is God himself. In those moments, while chewing the peyote, we must fall asleep concentrating on our Internal God. The exact outcome will be the astral projection. Then we will travel in the Astral Body. This is how we will be able to see, hear, and touch the things of the Ultra of Nature.

The things seen by the peyote are not hallucinations as the ignorant people believe. The intellectuals know that a fourth dimension exists. Any educated person knows this. Science has demonstrated that the perception of our five senses is very limited. Beneath the color red is found the gamma of the infrared; above the color violet is found the gamma of the ultraviolet. Science does not ignore this. The loss of elasticity in the crystalline (lens of the eye) prevents the image from forming in the retina. This is what is called bad focusing. In reality, no one perceives the object in itself, but merely the image of the object. Short-sightedness prevents us from seeing the image of a faraway object. There also exists Daltonism. The inflammation of the retina causes Daltonism; this is the confusion of colors.

In conclusion, the human eye only perceives sensible images. That is all.

However, Ultra-sensible images in the Ultra, and senses conditioned to receive those images also exist. Those senses enter into activity with the peyote. This is how we perceive the images of the Ultra.

Therefore, if those images of the Ultra were hallucinations, as the ignorant people say, then the sensible images that form in the retina would also be hallucinations.

We need to let go of eighteenth century materialism. We need to be more analytic, less dogmatic, and more didactic.

Matter is condensed energy. Energy condenses into different states. Factually, there exist masses whose grade of energetic vibration is so fast that their sensible images escape our five senses' perception.

Likewise, there exist masses in which the grade of vibration is so slow that they submerge beneath the limits of our sensorial perception.

Physical masses that the human being is normally incapable of perceiving exist above and below the limits of our external sensorial perception. Only with the powers of our Astral Body can we perceive other dimensions of the universe and life.

The peyote has the power to put into activity, even if it is momentary, those wonderful faculties that allow us to investigate the fourth dimension of Nature.

Many people might state that they do not believe. However, this is not a subject matter to believe or not to believe. These are scientific matters that need logical analysis and scientific investigation, free of prejudices and fanaticism. It needs experimentation.

One must explore profoundly all the recondite parts of the human being. We must not confine ourselves inside intransigent scientific dogmatisms. We need to be more liberal in our analysis. Materialism has already failed in Soviet Russia. The failure of materialism is proven by the fact that fifteen million Muslims exist in Russia.

The perceptions of the Ultra are as natural as the perceptions of the five ordinary senses. These are not hallucinating deliriums as the ignorant people believe. This is not about convulsive pathologic suggestions from ignorant, fanatic, hallucinated people. We need more study and less pride. The perceptions of the Ultra exist and must be studied.

The uncivilized natives in the Republic of Haiti who practice voodoo can be criticized because of their practices of black magic and because of their lack of intellectual culture. Yet indeed, we do not have the scientific basis of any kind to judge with all logical preciseness their hypersensible perceptions.

We do not deny that in many psychics exist psychic paroxysms accompanied by convulsions, pythonism with all its manifestations etc., etc. The pythonic crisis, the so called crisis of Loa of the Haitians, the ecstatic-convulsive crises during which they have super-sensible perception, are in depth absolutely unknown to science and forensic psychiatry.

If we put aside our intellectual pride, we will arrive at the conclusion that we can analyze sensible phenomena, objective states of the human organism. However, conventional science still has no authority in order to judge in a total form the perceptions of the Ultra.

With no doubt, fanaticism is the worst enemy of reasoning and logic; however, people from universities also fall into fanaticism.

When people from the universities laugh at clairvoyants and at convulsive-ecstatic crisis, when we believe that all the visions that are seen during one of those crisis are hallucinations, madness, etc., etc., by dint of pride, we fall into the state of fanaticism and ignorance. Our fanaticism is hallucinated by the theories that we have read and by the intellectual principles with which we mold our intellect.

If we believe that others are ignorant, likewise they may categorize us as ignorant, even if we believe that we are very cultured.

We are not the masters of knowledge. Therefore, convulsive and pathologic intellectual suggestion can convert an intellectual into an intolerable fanatic.

Many natives of Haiti who practice voodoo perceive with their clairvoyance tremendous realities of the Ultra of Nature. In order to discuss something, it is necessary to know about it. Therefore, the opinion of a critic has no value whatsoever if he has not a complete knowledge of the subject matter. People from universities do not practiced voodoo; they do not know it. Therefore, they do not have a complete knowledge of the subject matter.

People from universities see the natives of Haiti in their pythonismic crisis. Yet, they do not know anything about the things that those natives see in their trances, because people from university have not gone through those famous pythonic crises. The only thing they can do is to launch opinions without basis, because they have no complete knowledge of the case.

The prostatic chakra grants to every human being the power to project himself into the Astral Body consciously. The important thing is to develop this chakra.

We repeat, this is not a subject matter to believe or not to believe. The important thing is to study, analyze, and experience.

When any intellectual person states, “I do not believe in that,” they are demonstrating that they are superstitious. A cultured, studious, and investigative person states, “I will study it. I will experience it. I will analyze it.”

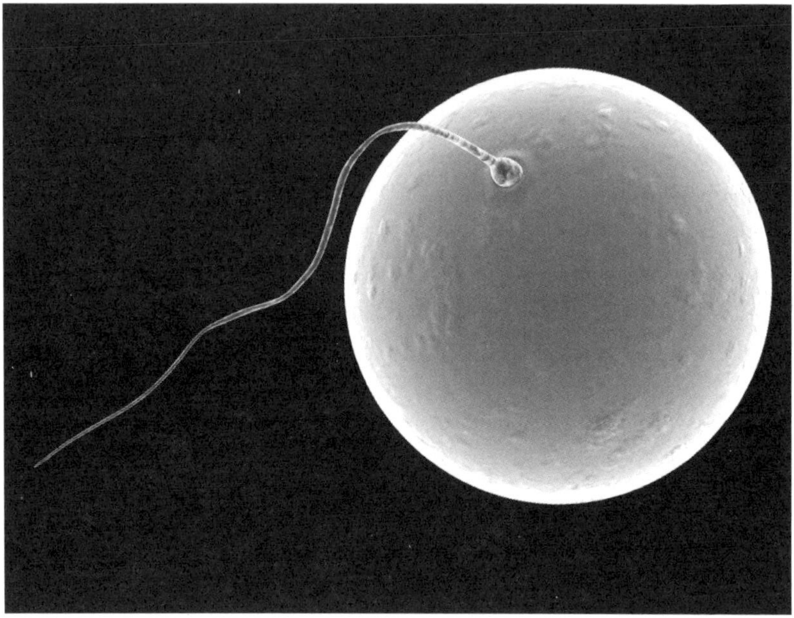

The Cosmic Consciousness is the primary intelligence that establishes the union of the spermatozoon with the ovum.

Chapter 14

The Testicles and the Ovaries

The internal secretions of the testicles and the ovaries are definitive for the life of the human being on the Earth. The fundamental differences between men and women are due to the secretions of the testicles and the ovaries.

Only one spermatozoon and one ovum are necessary for the reproduction of the human species. That is all. Therefore, scientifically, we do not see the reason why the male enjoys spilling millions of spermatozoa, when indeed only one is needed to fecundate.

The egg is big, round and possesses its own nucleus with a thick protoplasm that has an aspect of a yolk.

The spermatozoon is different; it is long and slim, has a pointed and oval body where the fundamental nucleus is found. The spermatozoon has a long tail resembling a tadpole.

The movement of the feminine egg within the waters of life is slow. The feminine egg waits patiently for the masculine spermatozoon to find it. The male's spermatozoon, propelling itself with its fish tail within the waters of the sexual chaos, navigates very far in search of the egg that awaits it.

The biologists do not know with scientific exactitude the *causa causorum* that unites the spermatozoon to the egg. For science, this is an enigma. As in everything, scientists launch hypotheses which are more or less their scientific opinions. Thus, it is believed that the protoplasm of the egg possesses a great chemical attraction to the sperm, etc., etc. All these are hypotheses but nothing more than hypotheses! Even if this hypothesis were to be true, it would still not resolve the enigma.

We cannot logically admit that a chemical reaction can be performed by itself without a conscious, controlling principle.

From the protoplasm of the egg, we will go on to the energetics of the egg.

Logic invites us to accept energy as a magnetic field of attraction to the egg. Logic invites us to accept electricity as a dynamic force impelling the spermatozoon to the egg.

In the final synthesis, the atom is an exponent of energies. The electromagnetic forces of every protoplasm are a tremendous reality. Everything radiates. We admit the mechanics of the phenomena, yet we need an explanation of the laws that regulate such mechanics.

Indeed, the Cosmic Consciousness is the primary intelligence that establishes the union of the spermatozoon with the ovum. We cannot accept an intelligent phenomenon without an intelligent cause. Facts are facts and before the facts we must surrender.

Gnostics talk about the Third Logos. Science must know that the Third Logos is that primary intelligence. The Third Logos is not an individual. The Third Logos of the Gnostics is the primary intelligence of Nature.

The creative energy of the Third Logos is that primary intelligence of Nature that unites the spermatozoon with the ovum. The creative energy of the Third Logos bipolarizes itself into positive and negative.

The spermatozoon is the exponent of the positive forces of the Third Logos. The ovum is the exponent of the negative forces of the Third Logos. Both poles of the energies unite in order to create. The Law is the Law.

The decapitation of John the Baptist occurs when the spermatozoon enters the ovum.

The materialist partisans of Darwinism point out the similarities of all animals in the embryonic state, including the human being. This they do in order to prove that the more complex and superior species have emerged by evolution and transformation from the more simple and inferior species.

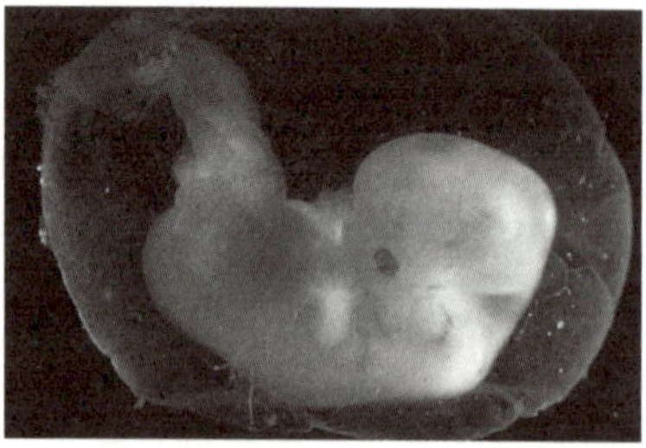
THE HUMAN EMBRYO AT FIVE WEEKS OLD

Nonetheless, we, the Gnostics, consider that the similarities of the animals in their embryonic state, including the human being, are revealing to satiety two things: first, the unity of life, second, an original genetic seed.

The seed of all that exists sleeps as an original seed within the seminal atoms of the Grand Universal Life.

The creative energy of the Third Logos makes the waters of life, the universal semen, to become fecund. This is how the germs of every existence sprout.

Every species has a universal prototype within the original chaos. In the famous blastoderm, three layers of absolutely different cells exist. The first one is the internal, the second one is middle, and the third one is the external.

The spermatozoon united with the ovum multiplies by cellular division; this is how that cellular community called the blastoderm is created.

The gelatinous state of the spermatozoon and the ovum demonstrate that in the beginning of the universe, life was subtle, fluidic and gelatinous, and afterwards more gross and hard. This reminds us of the great turtle worshipped by the Mayan Indians. First, it is subtle and gelatinous, afterwards appears its hard shell full of constellations and worlds. As above so below... Fortunately, the scientists in Russia have discovered worlds in a protoplasmic state.

The spermatozoon and the ovum must pass through a process of evolution and development before becoming a new vehicle for the human soul. The internal causes for the maturation of the ovum-sperm are very unknown to biology.

The intimate causes for the maturation of a universe in a protoplasmic state are an enigma to astronomy and astrophysics.

It would be very interesting if the scientists would resolve the enigma of the chromosomes. Why does the egg have only 48 chromosomes? Why does the spermatozoon also have 48 chromosomes? Enigmas! Enigmas! Enigmas!

What is the intimate motive for the spermatozoon and the ovum during their maturation to lose exactly the same mathematical number of 24 chromosomes each? Who is the one who endures the inconvenience of making such a perfect mathematical calculation?

For what reasons when a spermatozoon united with an ovum after their maturation do they together come to have the same original number of 48 chromosomes?

Two mathematical operations exist in this, namely: subtraction and addition. The basic capital is 48. Can mathematical operations exist without a mathematical intelligence? All of this is showing us through simple logical deduction the reality of the primary intelligence of nature that we, the Gnostics, call the Third Logos.

After the human spermatozoon has fecundated the human ovum, the uterus gestates for nine months.

The cell of the ovum and sperm has two nuclei - one from the sperm and the other from the ovum. These two nuclei join themselves wisely. The protoplasm of both nuclei mixes among themselves.

A sphere of attraction exists inside the ovum-sperm cell. The great sphere of attraction also bipolarizes, obeying the primary intelligence. Each one of the two polarities of that sphere of attraction contracts and expands the nucleus, converting it into the mitotic spindle.

The chromosomes and genes are found mixed within the center of the nuclei mitotic spindle. The genes are inside the chromosomes. The genes give us the heredity of our father and mother.

Nevertheless, not everything that the human being receives is hereditary. Terrible murderers have been born from virtuous families and great geniuses have been born from mediocre families.

If a clairvoyant examines an already mature spermatozoon when it directs itself into the ovum, then the clairvoyant will see in the superior vortex of the spermatozoon a very important atom. This is the Seed Atom. This atom is a trio of matter, energy, and consciousness. A very fine thread that is united to a certain sum of energetic values of Nature comes from that atom. Those values are related to the soul, to the Being.

We are, within the space, points who accede to serve as vehicles of determined sums of values from Nature. Therefore, death is just a subtraction of fractions. Once the subtraction (death) is done, only those values remain.

Those values of Nature are electromagnetic. Once the physical body is dead, those values rebuild another one through new biological processes, whose steps are followed very carefully by biology. This is the law of reincorporation. The law is the law, and the law is fulfilled.

Energy exists inside the physical atoms of the ovum-sperm. This energy forms the Mumia. The atoms of the Astral Body abide inside each atom of the Mumia. We know Theosophy's septuple constitution of the human being; however, here we are just synthesizing.

We are not setting down dogmas. We are analyzing. Science has already been capable of the materialization of the Astral Body in some laboratories. Facts are facts, and before the facts, we must surrender.

The virtues and defects of every human being depend upon the quality of values that reincarnate in them. For instance, a dervish Moor who studied the Koran lived in Spain during the era of the Moorish dominion over Spain. He read the Koran and studied the Bible. The outcome was that the knowledge ingested in him, and he became full of skepticism. That dervish Moor died full of doubts. At a later date, the values from that dervish Moor reincorporated and became a man named Voltaire.

Any human being can develop clairvoyance and see the values of the consciousness evolving throughout space and time.

The great American physiologist Brown-Sequard, mentioned by Dr. Krumm-Heller, invented a system of healing that was judged by many people as immoral. This system consists on exciting the sexual organ without reaching the orgasm and the spilling of the semen. In this case, the semen is cerebrated and the cerebrum is semenized. Thus the semen is assimilated inside the organism and the nervous system nourishes and fortifies itself totally. This system would not be an obstacle for the reproduction of the species. A spermatozoon can easily escape from the organism without the necessity of spilling millions of spermatozoa that are lost in a seminal ejaculation.

The system of Brown-Sequard is known in Italy as Karezza. This is the **Arcanum A.Z.F.**

Dr. Krumm-Heller stated that impotence can be cured with this system.

On page 174 of the *Rosicrucian Novel*, Dr. Krumm-Heller states the following:

> "The Rosicrucian Studies teach us that the semen is the astral liquid of the human being; it is life; it encloses power. Yet, it is so immense a power, that knowing how to drive it, one can achieve everything. This is why it is so important to know the Rosicrucian Secrets, because one possesses a powerful weapon against the adversities of destiny."

On page 172 of the same novel, Dr. Krumm-Heller states the following:

> "The Rosicrucian magician feels the same nervous arousing as any human being full of desire. If men would know what they are capable of doing during this moment of nervousness, I am sure they would do anything but to follow the woman."

The Aztec sages of ancient Mexico knew very well what can be done in that moment of nervousness. Men and women remained naked inside the stony patios of the Aztec Temples; there they were loving each other, uniting themselves sexually for months.

Those couples knew how to withdraw from the sexual act before the orgasm. This is how they avoided the ejaculation of their semen. These couples did not allow the wonderful semen to escape out of their organism. This is the famous Italian Karezza, the system of the great American Brown-Sequard.

The awakening of the Kundalini is achieved with Brown-Sequard's system. Indeed, surgeons will not be able to find the Kundalini with the surgical scalpel. Yet, if they were to practice the Gnostic-Rosicrucian exercises, then they would become clairvoyant. Any clairvoyant doctor can see the Kundalini.

The Kundalini is the Aztec Serpent Quetzacoatl; that is, the fire of the Holy Spirit, the Igneous Serpent of our Magical Powers.

The clairvoyant Yogi sees a lotus flower with four wonderful petals situated exactly between the sexual organs and the anus.

This lotus flower with four wonderful petals is the church of Ephesus, the Muladhara chakra. The Kundalini is found inside this chakra. The Kundalini has the shape of a sacred serpent; it is a solar spiritual fiery serpent that can only be seen with clairvoyance. It cannot be found with the surgical scalpel because it is not material.

The Kundalini is concentrated Akasha. Akasha is the cause of Ether and the agency of sound. Only those who raise the Akasic Serpent through the *canalis centralis* of the spinal medulla can incarnate the Word.

The Kundalini develops, evolves, and progresses inside the aura of the Solar Logos.

The chakra of the sexual organs is the center of the Prithvi Tattva (the Petrous Ether). Whosoever controls the Prithvi Tattva can control earthquakes.

Seven magnetic centers exist within the spinal medulla. These seven centers of the spinal medulla are connected with the seven important plexus of the Grand Sympathetic Nervous System. All the Tattvic powers are within those seven centers. The flaming Akasha opens those seven Tattvic centers of the spinal medulla. This is how we become masters of the Tattvas.

1. The first magnetic center of the spinal medulla is the abode of the Tattva Prithvi, the power of sex.

2. The second one corresponds to the Prostatic (Uterine) chakra. This is the church of the Tattva Apas (Water), liquid Ether.

3. The third chakra is at the height of the navel. It is related to the solar plexus. This is the church of the Tattva Tejas (Igneous Ether), universal fire.

4. The fourth center of the spinal medulla corresponds to the chakra of the heart. This is the sacred abode of the Tattva Vayu (Gaseous Ether). These are the four inferior Tattvic centers of the human temple.

The tower of the temple is the neck and the head. The following three superior Tattvic centers exist in this human tower.

5. The fifth center is the larynx. This is the church of the Word. Sound cannot exist without Akasha. The Kundalini becomes creative with the Word.

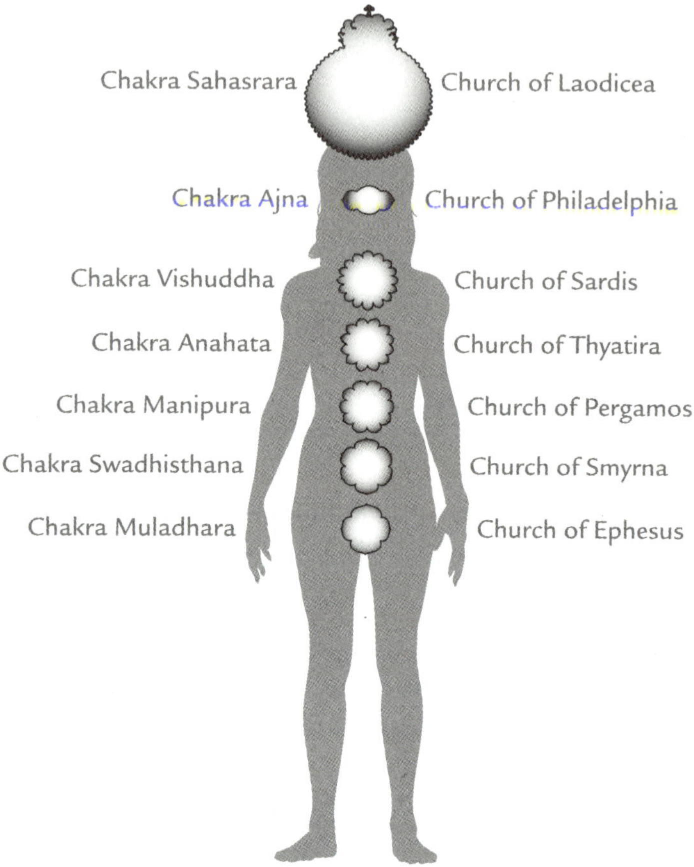

THE SEVEN PRIMARY CHAKRAS OR CHURCHES

6. The sixth magnetic center is related with the frontal chakra. This is the center of clairvoyance. When the Kundalini opens this center the human being becomes clairvoyant. This is how one can see the Ultra.

7. The seventh Tattvic center is the chakra of the thousand petals situated in the pineal gland. When the Kundalini opens this chakra we receive polyvoyance, omniscience, etc.

We receive all these powers with the system of Brown-Sequard. The only requisite is never to spill the semen during our whole life. Brown-Sequard's system is the **Arcanum A.Z.F.**

The famous North American Kabbalist Manly P. Hall, mentioned by the Dr. Francis A. Propato, states in his book *Occult Anatomy* the following, "Those who are incapable of raising the fire of the spinal medulla through their sushumna channel will be cast down into a lateral kingdom similar to that of today's apes (monkeys, gorillas, etc.)." The sushumna channel runs lengthwise and inwards within the medullar canal.

The Arcanum A.Z.F. must only be practiced between husband and wife in legitimately constituted homes.

Those men who practice the Arcanum A.Z.F. with many women commit the serious crime of adultery. The adulterous man will never achieve the awakening of the Kundalini and the Tattvic powers.

Likewise will happen with women; the adulterous woman who practices the Arcanum A.Z.F. with many men will never awaken the Kundalini or the Tattvic powers.

The Gnostic Initiates who adulterate loose their powers.

God is the Innermost. God is the Inner Being of each human being who comes to the world. God is a divine Hermaphrodite, Male-Female. God does not need a spouse to light the fire. Yet, the human being is not God. Human beings cannot light their fires without a spouse. The human being needs a spouse to enlighten the fires, because the human being is not God.

The human being must put aside the pride of believing that he is a God, because the human being is nothing more than a miserable slug that wallows in the mud of the earth.

The great female yogi Helena Petrovna Blavatsky, after becoming the widow of the Count Blavatsky, had to remarry again with Colonel Olcott in order to awaken her Kundalini and achieve the Tattvic powers.

The Sacred Order of Tibet teaches their disciples the Arcanum A.Z.F.

In the mysteries of Egypt, the Arcanum A.Z.F. was taught to the Initiates, and those who would divulge this great Arcanum were condemned to death. They were taken to a patio, and there, against a wall, they were decapitated. Their hearts were stripped away and their ashes were thrown to the four winds.

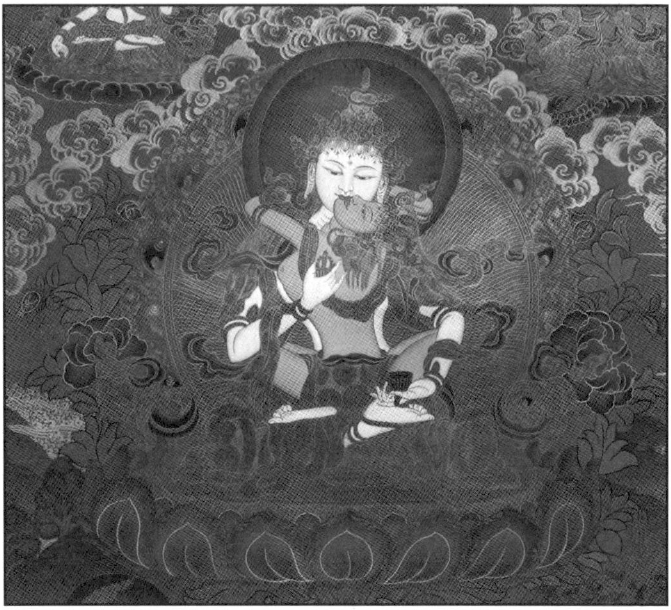

THE PRACTICE OF KARMA MUDRA AS DEPICTED IN TIBETAN TANTRISM

There was never known within any school of mysteries someone who had achieved initiation without the Great Arcanum A.Z.F.

Men and women remained naked, participating in the Arcanum A.Z.F. for entire months within the patios of the Temple of the Aztecs. Whosoever that by any chance ejaculated the semen was condemed to death for profaning the Temple. Afterwards, he was decapitated.

The Initiates from the schools of mystery of all times received initiations with the Great Arcanum. There was never known within any school of mysteries someone who had achieved initiation without the Great Arcanum A.Z.F. This is the Great Arcanum.

Once, on a given occasion, after having dictated a lecture, a bachelor disciple asked us if it were possible to practice the Great Arcanum with a woman of the Astral World. We answered him that only with a woman of flesh and blood is it possible to awaken Kundalini.

Another brother who was also a bachelor wanted to practice with imaginary women! This is very ominous! When the mind creates a mental effigy, this effigy acquires consciousness and converts itself into a tempting demon of the Mental World. During sleep, this effigy discharges us sexually through nocturnal pollutions (wet dreams).

It is very difficult for a student to disintegrate those mental effigies. Commonly, the students become victims of those mental effigies that their own mind invented. The best is to find a spouse that will really cooperate in the Grand Opus.

Those who do not have a spouse must raise their creative energy with sports in the open air, like hiking excursions and swimming. They must raise their creative energy when listening to good music and when admiring the great works of art: sculpture, painting, classical music, etc.

In this way, the unmarried ones can raise their sexual energies and bring them up toward their hearts. There in that center of life those creative forces mix themselves with the luminous waves of the Internal Christ and are taken toward the ineffable regions of the Great Light. We also elevate the sexual energies with the aesthetic sense, with charity, and love.

Nevertheless, in the name of Truth, we must affirm the following: If you want the higher initiation, if you long for the awakening of the Kundalini and the Tattvic powers, you need to find a spouse, because the Initiate without a spouse is like a garden without water.

Many mystical Initiates believe that they are chaste because they do not have a spouse. Nevertheless, they have nocturnal pollutions. This is how they miserably loose their Christic semen, within which is found the Genesis of the Great Life.

The sacred fire of the Solar Logos (Christ) is found within every seed, whether it is vegetable, animal, or human seed. This is why the seed has the power to reproduce itself.

Human beings must take care of their semen, their seed, as if it was potable gold.

We heroically extract the sacred fire of the Kundalini from our seed through the Arcanum A.Z.F.

Nocturnal pollutions are radically healed with the Arcanum A.Z.F.

We are children of a man and a woman. We are not children of any theory. The Word, the Son of Man, is the child of a man and a woman. The Son of Man is the child of Immaculate Conceptions. We need to lift up the Son of Man inside ourselves, and in order to lift up the Son of Man inside ourselves we need a spouse.

Part II
Criminology

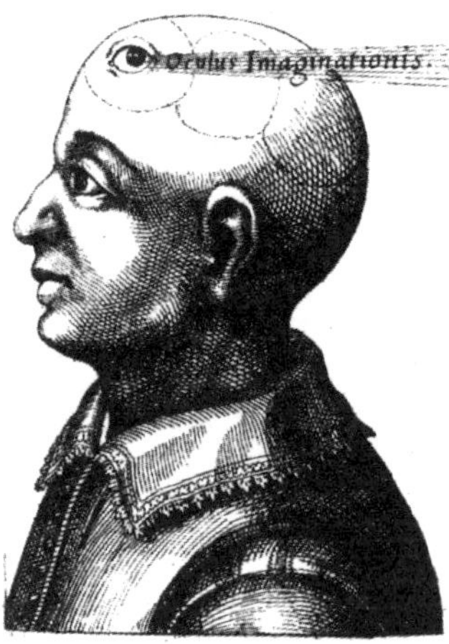

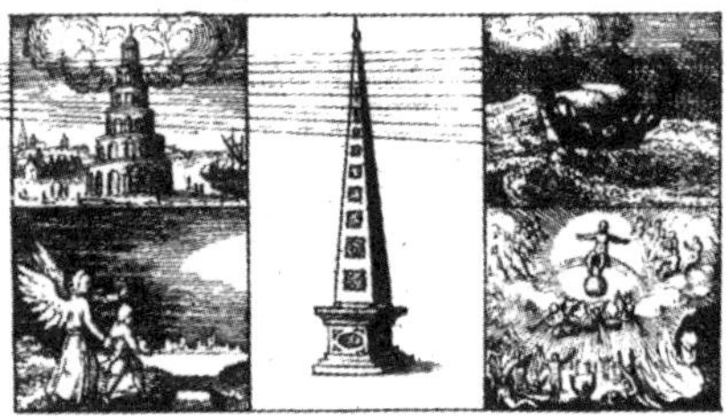

ENGRAVING BY ROBERT FLUDD

Clairvoyance: (French)
clair-: clear; -voyance: vision.

Clairvoyance is Imagination. Imagination can be positive (conscious imagination) or negative (fantasy, or mechanical imagination).

Conscious imagination is the clear means through which is reflected the firmament, the mysteries of life and death and of the Being. Mechanical imagination is different. It is formed by the debris of the memory, and it is fantasy.
- Samael Aun Weor

Chapter 15

Different Types of Clairvoyant Perception

There exist five types of fundamental clairvoyant perceptions.

1. Conscious clairvoyance
2. Unconscious clairvoyance
3. Infraconscious clairvoyance
4. Subconscious clairvoyance
5. Supraconscious clairvoyance

These five types of clairvoyant perceptions produce different forms of mental reactions.

Different biotypological characters exist in forensic psychiatry.

Diagnostically speaking, when receiving the impact of clairvoyant perceptions, each personality reacts in accordance to their particular, individual psycho-pathology.

There exists the apparantly "normal" paranoid, and the ill paranoid. There also exists the schizophrenic with violent, instantaneous, and terrible reactions. There also exists the neurasthenic with an ill double personality, the assassin and vulgar oligophrenic, the epileptic, the hypersensible type of schizoid or hyper-aesthetic with epileptic genotype, etc., etc.

During the moment of a conditional reaction, every clairvoyant speaks and acts conditioned by the type of psychopathological pesonality that characterizes him as a human entity.

For the development of clairvoyance, it is necessary to possess an intellectual culture. To have an intellectual discipline is necessary for the development of the latent powers, chakras, discs, magnetic wheels of the Astral Body.

A clairvoyant without any intellectual culture and without any intellectual discipline degenerates into a delinquent and vulgar person. A clairvoyant without any intellectual culture can fall into the following crimes: calumny, public or private slander, defamation of honor, threats, uxoricide, homicide, suicide, patricide, fratricide, incest, theft, matricide, kidnapping, ambush, sexual seduction, violence and force, infanticide, etc., etc., etc., and many other cases of crime studied by psychiatry and psychology.

The pathogenic role of the superstitious fear induced by the infraconscious, subconscious, or unconscious clairvoyant perceptions give origin to murder, calumny, and public slander, and in general to all kinds of common crimes. The infraconscious, subconscious, or unconscious clairvoyant perceptions produce different situational reactions in accordance with the biotypological type of clairvoyant.

The different types of clairvoyants, namely the neurasthenic, schizophrenic, oligophrenic, epileptic, and hypersensible class of schizoid, fall into states of psychopathic consternation, compulsive and pathological suggestion, superstitious delirium of persecution, etc. All of these take them into the abyss of delinquency.

Therefore, before delivering ourselves to the development of occult powers, we need to study ourselves and make a personological, psychopathological diagnosis of our own personality.

After discovering our own particular psychobiotypological "I" we need to reform ourselves with an intellectual culture. We need a pedagogic psychotherapy in order to reform ourselves.

Indeed, the four gospels of Jesus Christ are the best pedagogic psychotherapy. It is necessary to totally study and practice all the teachings contained in the four gospels of Jesus Christ.

Therefore, only after reforming ourselves morally can we deliver ourselves to the development of the chakra discs, magnetic wheels, of the Astral Body. It is also urgent to study the best authors of Theosophy, Rosicrucianism, Psychology, Yoga, etc., etc.

Chapter 16

Positive and Negative Clairvoyance

The Rosicrucian Initiate Max Heindel states in his book *The Rosicrucian Cosmo-conception* that when the chakras of the Astral Body rotate from left to right (clockwise), then clairvoyance becomes positive. Max Heindel asseverates that when the chakras rotate from right to left (counterclockwise), then clairvoyance becomes negative.

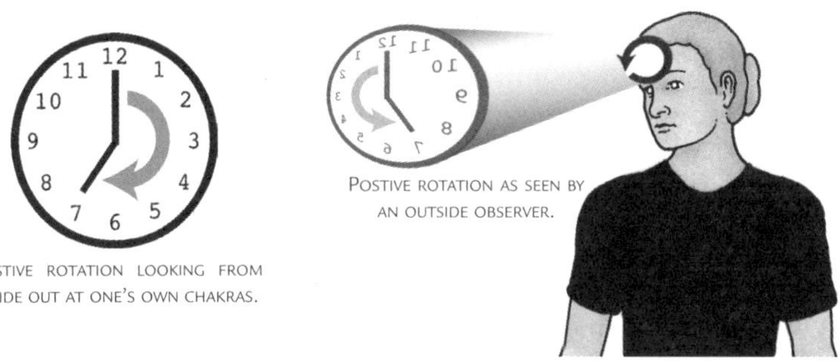

Observing from within one's own body, the positive rotation of the chakras is clockwise. The same rotation, observed from afar, appears counter-clockwise. The opposite rotation (i.e., negative) is what is commonly seen and taught.

The exerted clairvoyants are positive. The mediums and seers of Spiritism or Spiritualism are negative. The positive clairvoyant knows how to drive his faculty by will. The negative clairvoyant sees without wanting to see. The negative clairvoyant always becomes cheated by the tenebrous entities.

The crime of "Mama Coleta" that occurred February 6,1944 on the San Francisco Farm, Rodrigo neighborhood, close to Cifuentes, Province Las Villas, Cuba, is a concrete example of what negative clairvoyance is, as well as the Spiritist or Spiritualist mediumism.

The neighborhood of "Mama Coleta" was indeed the scenario for mediumism, spiritualism, negative clairvoyance, incest and crime.

The female Medium, Francisca, with her psychopathic and nervous personality, was indeed victim of the tenebrous entities that wander in the Astral Plane. The medium Francisca's fear contaminated her sister Candida. The two sisters sheltered themselves in the bed of their brother Candido. This is how both sisters fell into the crime of incest. There was a double incest.

Their brother Candido had lived with a concubine; thus, when he saw the nervous state of his clairvoyant sister, he distrusted the woman with whom he had lived. He supposed that his ex-concubine had cast a spell to their home. The panic reached the maximum when his younger brother brought him a doll that the ex-concubine had given him as a gift.

Afterwards, came the second part of this drama that culminated with the crime of "Mama Coleta." Candido consulted a "santero" who, in spite of the opposition of "Mama Coleta," performed some ceremonies and a cleanse onto the medium seer, Francisca. Thereafter, he declared that the one who was responsible for his disgrace was the soul of a warlock named Barrueta.

Afterwards, the "santero" granted onto the medium seer Francisca the power of rejecting spells. Indeed, the female medium, Francisca, with her negative clairvoyance, was seeing the tenebrous entities. She was seeing against her will. She was seeing demons everywhere. She could not control her sixth sense.

When "Mama Coleta" discovered the incest, the negative clairvoyant Francisca defended herself by stating that she did not have carnal relations with her brother. She was instead having intercourse with the soul of the warlock Barrueta, who was inserting himself within the body of her brother. To that end, in accordance with her, she was not perpetrating the crime of incest.

The night of the events was terrible. The medium Francisca seemed a lunatic. She violently ejected the food that was cooked for her, believing it to be poisoned. She ripped at the furniture of her home. She threw the clothes of her family outside their house. She was in a state of delirium: shouting, dancing, and clairvoyantly seeing the warlock Barrueta.

Her whole family kneeled with their faces towards a wall with their arms opened in the shape of the cross. Soon, all of them fell into a mass suggestion. All of her brothers struck the father of that family, because they stated that the warlock Barrueta was inserted within the body of their father.

Afterwards, they killed "Mama Coleta" by punching her horribly, because the seer Francisca saw the demons going inside the body of the wretched old woman.

The last victim of the negative clairvoyance of that medium was her brother. The seer Francisca saw her brother transforming himself into the warlock Barrueta. Thus, she struck her brother's head with a big heavy rock that fractured the bones of his cranium and tossed out from it pieces of his encephalic mass.

The last thing that this female seer did, naked and armed with a stick, was ride a horse outside in the streets. Screaming around the streets, she was riding the horse while beating around demons with the stick. Moments after, she was stopped by the police and everything ended when all of them were imprisoned.

The former narrative is a concrete case of what negative clairvoyance is. The seer Francisca had a "mental deficit, together with transitory amnesia and absolutely negative clairvoyant visions of a mediumistic character."

Commonly, these types of seers are oligophrenics who exhibit the same credibility as a weak and thoughtless being.

These negative seers fall into compulsive suggestion. These negative seers, while under their compulsive or pathologic suggestion, reach the horrible abyss of delinquency.

Indeed, these negative clairvoyants see forms that exist within the infraconsciousness of this great Nature.

A true scientist cannot accept as infallible the visions of a negative clairvoyant. Only true, positive clairvoyance is infallible.

In order to develop positive clairvoyance, it is required to practice the necessary esoteric exercises and to study the best authors of Theosophy, Rosicrucianism, Yoga, Psychology, etc., etc.

Our worst enemy is ignorance; therefore, we recommend our readers study the great works of the female Master Helena Petrovna Blavatsky, entitled *The Secret Doctrine.* We also recommend *Kundalini Yoga* of Sivananda, the books of Dr. Arnold Krumm-Heller, the books of Dr. Adoum, the books of Rudolf Steiner, etc., etc.

Positive clairvoyance is achieved only with a great intellectual culture and a great esoteric discipline. The highest cultured people, who are submitted to the most rigorous intellectual disciplines, only achieve the truly positive clairvoyance. The illuminated intellect is the outcome of positive clairvoyance.

Chapter 17

The Consciousness

Only those who have achieved the awakening in the superior worlds possess **Conscious Clairvoyance**.

During the normal hours of sleep, all human beings wrapped in their Astral Bodies live in the suprasensible worlds.

Humanity lives during sleep and after death in the suprasensible regions of the great Mother Nature. Unfortunately, people act with their consciousness asleep while in the suprasensible worlds.

Positive clairvoyance is possessed only by the souls who live awakened in the suprasensible worlds. Indeed, those who possess Continuous Consciousness, whether out of their body when it is asleep or inside it when it is awake, are always in the state of watchfulness. They are positive clairvoyants. They possess Continuous Consciousness.

Every authentic extrasensory or esoteric investigation departs from that perfect state of surveillance.

It is necessary for the dreamer to awaken within the internal worlds before converting himself into a competent investigator in the superior worlds.

The mediums of spiritism or spiritualism are incompetent to investigate in the superior worlds, because they have their Mental Body dislocated. The mediums of spiritualism are mentally unbalanced; therefore, any investigation they attempt to do in the superior worlds results in failure.

The psychopathic states of the mediums of spiritualism, the compulsive and pathologic suggestions, the paroxysmal epileptic states during their trance, and the psychic obsession to which they are exposed, convert them into fallacious, abnormal and mentally unbalanced individuals.

Logical thought and exact concepts are necessary in order to investigate in the superior worlds.

Every true, positive vision must be totally supported by concrete facts of the physical world.

The truth does not diverge from human nature. Therefore, if what we consider true diverges from human nature, then it cannot be true.

If the clairvoyant is not a saint, then at least he must be a perfect gentleman.

We know of the case of a paranoid clairvoyant who slandered a virtuous mother, accusing her publicly and pointing her out as an adulterer and a witch, etc., etc. This poor innocent and virtuous woman was mocked publicly by the paranoid clairvoyant. We also know about another case where the clairvoyant was a neurasthenic; he slandered and threatened to death a virtuous and honorable citizen accusing him of being a warlock and asseverating that he was endowed with diabolic powers.

We know about a schizophrenic clairvoyant who reacted instantaneously against an honorable citizen. The schizophrenic clairvoyant accused that man of having an affair with the clairvoyant's wife. The schizophrenic clairvoyant said that he saw this with the use of his clairvoyance. If this clairvoyant had been a neurasthenic, he would have murdered that gentleman. If he had been paranoid, he would have studied and planned a perfect murder. If he had been an oligophrenic, he would have killed the man by starving him or by shooting him, even though the victim had never thought of having an affair with the clairvoyant's wife.

If the clairvoyant had declared his accusation in front of the judges, they would have declared the other man innocent because of the lack of evidence, since in order to sentence someone it is necessary to prove the "corpus delicti," the responsibility of the accused.

The majority of clairvoyants could be prosecuted for slander, threats, and defamation of character.

Another aspect that one must take into account is the evidence of the "corpus delicti." If the "corpus delicti" is not demonstrated in any of the established forms and penal code proceedings, then the accused is innocent.

Therefore all things whatsoever ye would that men should do to you, do ye even so to them.

MATTHEW 7:12

> *The truth does not diverge from human nature. Therefore, if what we consider true diverges from human nature, then it cannot be true.*

Christ said:

> *Judge not, that ye be not judged. For with what judgment ye judge, ye shall be judged and with what measure ye mete, it shall be measured to you again.*
>
> Matthew 7:1, 2

The clairvoyant must be rigorously analytic, highly intellectual and strictly scientific.

The clairvoyant's worst enemy is **ignorance**. The clairvoyant must learn to see in the absence of the "I," the myself. The clairvoyant must see without judging.

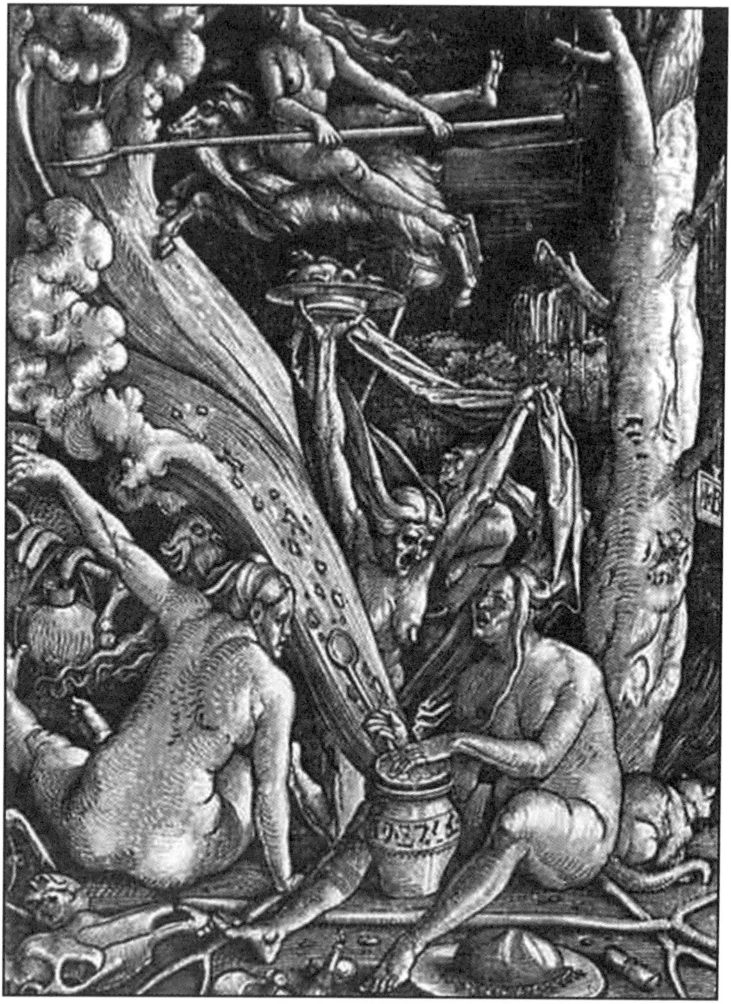

The Witches' Sabbath with its black masses and its witchcraft were in rivalry with the Priests of the "holy office" of the Catholic Inquisition in regards to the assassination of innocent children. This is what sadomasochist clairvoyance is, a criminal and terribly perverse type of clairvoyance.

Chapter 18

The Psycho-bio-typic "I"

The mind is bottled up within the "I." Every conditional reaction of the mind is the outcome of the psycho-bio-typic "I."

Every perception passes from the senses into the mind.

The "I" translates all the information that is collected by the mind in accordance with its own prejudices, desires, fears, remembrances, preconceptions, maliciousness of a certain type, fanaticism, hatred, envy, jealousy, passion, etc., etc.

The clairvoyant always has a bad secretary from whom he needs to liberate himself. This secretary is the "I," the *myself*, the ego.

The "I" of the clairvoyant traps all the suprasensible representations that arrive into his mind, then he interprets them in accordance with his prejudices, hatreds, jealousies, mistrusts, maliciousness of a certain type, passions, remembrances, pride, envy, arrogance, etc., etc. The subsequent reactions of the clairvoyant are the outcome of his own psycho-bio-typic "I."

The **paranoid** clairvoyant is full of pride. He likes to keep himself isolated from the world. He prefers to deal only with very few people. He is a very intelligent person, yet he is sly and distrustful. He tends to believe himself to be infallible. He believes himself to be a great Master. He believes that he can dominate the world. He does not accept opinions from anyone, since he believes that only he is truly wise, great, and powerful.

When this type of paranoid clairvoyant reacts with hatred, malice, distrust, etc., he can even, in cold blood, plan an Intellectual Assassination.

The **neurasthenic** clairvoyant has a double personality. Just as he prays and preaches ineffable things, he also speaks of pistols, daggers, war, violence, etc., etc. While in front of an unpleasant representation, this type of clairvoyant reacts with calumnies, insults, homicides, etc. When one of his two personalities becomes full of complexes or humiliated, he then asks for forgiveness and speaks with devotion in order to make amends. Once he attains his purposes, his other personality reacts with pride, anger, arrogance, violence, treason, etc.

An in-depth analysis upon this double personality type takes us to the conclusion that Judas Iscariot was a type of neurasthenic clairvoyant. Judas was of a double personality, since in one moment he was following the Master and in another he was against the Master. He kissed the Master, and thereafter he betrayed him. He repented of his doing, and thereafter he committed suicide. This is how the neurasthenic type is.

The "I," the Myself, does not exist within Christ. Christ does not react against calumnies, slaps, mockeries, threats, whippings, etc., etc. Christ overwhelms because of His terrific serenity. Christ when crucified said only, *"Father, forgive them; for they know not what they do."* The "I" does not exist inside the Christ; this is why He neither reacts nor judges anybody. Christ is a perfect clairvoyant who knows how to see with comprehension, without judging, without translating, because He does not have the "I." Christ is the clairvoyant who sees, comprehends and knows. Christ is the Universal Spirit of Life incarnated inside Jesus of Nazareth.

The clairvoyant needs to learn how to contemplate the internal representations in the absence of the "I." The clairvoyant needs to see without judging, without translating, without pre-concepts, without fanaticism, without passion, etc., etc. The clairvoyant needs to be highly comprehensive.

When a **schizophrenic** clairvoyant reacts against an unpleasant representation, he can fall into the worst crimes, because of his violent, instantaneous and terrible reactions.

Commonly, a schizoaffective clairvoyant is woeful, melancholic, auto-concentrated, and introspective. He possesses melancholic ideas; he gets weary with any intellectual work, etc., etc. The schizoid clairvoyant, while in front of an unpleasant representation, if he is not rigorously analytic, can react by murdering others and thereafter committing suicide.

A **masochist** clairvoyant enjoys whipping himself while in the presence of his mystical representations or performing terrible penances to the death.

Clairvoyance demands logical thought and an exact concept.

One needs to have perfect mental equilibrium in order to be an exerted clairvoyant.

A clairvoyant with some psychic trauma can suffer serious mental disorders and can unconsciously create fatal images within the Mental World.

When a mentally disordered clairvoyant contemplates his own suprasensible creations, he can then receive a nervous, emotional shock. He can also receive a vertiginous impetus, or an unexpected and acute emotional rapture. All of these with certainty can take this clairvoyant into the abyss of crime. The psychic trauma is the outcome of a great moral pain, or a great frightening experience, or the loss of a beloved one, etc., etc.

The **sadomasochist** clairvoyant has reached such a state of sexual perversion that he is easily converted into a mystic-erotic assassin. The sadomasochist clairvoyant loves the sweet evilness and falls into the bloodiest phallic cults. The black masses of the Middle Ages with their naked women upon the altar and the assassination of innocent children are living examples of this tenebrous and fatal kind of clairvoyance.

The human sacrifices of all times and of all religions are the outcome of the sadomasochist clairvoyance. Those human sacrifices are living examples that show us what this type of sadomasochist clairvoyance is. So, the assassination of people on the altar for liturgical ritual purposes is nothing else than a barbaric sadomasochist clairvoyant custom.

The black mass with human sacrifices was celebrated in many medieval castles during the XV century. Marshall Gil de Retz in Tiffanges, France, had in his castle a church whose priest celebrated the black mass. Retz was accused of having assassinated two hundred children in his black masses. Catalina de Medici also celebrated black masses with the sacrifice of innocent children.

The Witches' Sabbath with its black masses and its witchcraft were in rivalry with the Priests of the "holy office" of the Catholic Inquisition in regards to the assassination of innocent children. This is what sadomasochist clairvoyance is, a criminal and terribly perverse type of clairvoyance.

Therefore, we can become perfect clairvoyants only by dissolving the Psycho-bio-typic "I," which everybody carries inside.

Chapter 19

The Human Mind

The brain has five fundamental parts:

1. The encephalon
2. The cerebrum
3. The midbrain
4. The medulla oblongata or hindbrain
5. The pons or breach

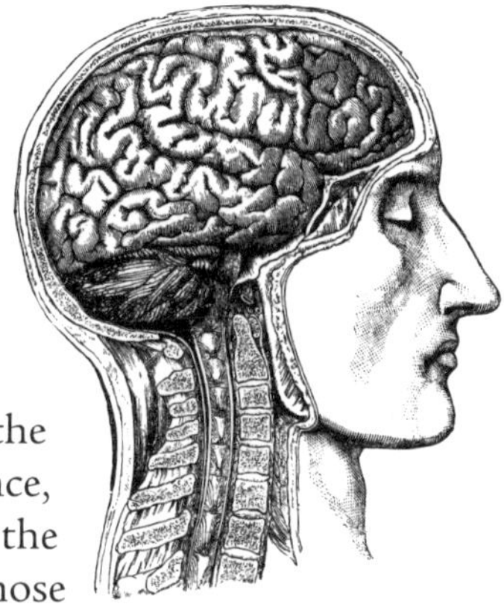

Indeed, those who state that the encephalon governs the intelligence, memory, willpower, etc., ignore the existence of the Mental Body. Those people should study all the volumes of *The Secret Doctrine* written by Helena Petrovna Blavatsky.

The brain is made in order to elaborate thought, yet it is not the thought. The brain is an instrument of the mind, yet it is not the mind. We must distinguish between the brain and the mind. We must study the intimate relations of the brain with the mind.

In our former chapters we spoke about the Astral Body. In those chapters we stated that the mind, the psychic and spiritual principles of the human being are within the Astral Body.

The mind is a subtle marvelous body that has its own Ultra-biology and Ultra-pathology that is in intimate relation with the Cerebrospinal Nervous System and the brain.

Thought is a function of the Mental Body. The human being can think without the physical brain; he can think independently without the aid of the cerebral matter. This has already been demonstrated in the scientific laboratories where some disincarnated entities were materialized.

We are stating concrete facts that are already demonstrated. If the reader still has not read anything about the materializations of Katie King in the laboratory of Sir William Crookes with the help of the Fox sisters, the mediums for materialization, then we recommend to do it. The concrete fact is that the Astral Body of the defunct Katie King was materializing itself throughout three consecutive years in the already mentioned scientific laboratory. Then, the scientists saw, heard, touched, etc., etc. the entity. Katie King allowed herself to be submitted to all types of experiments. Frauds did not happen there, because the scientists controlled the experiments to prevent even the slightest possibility of fraud.

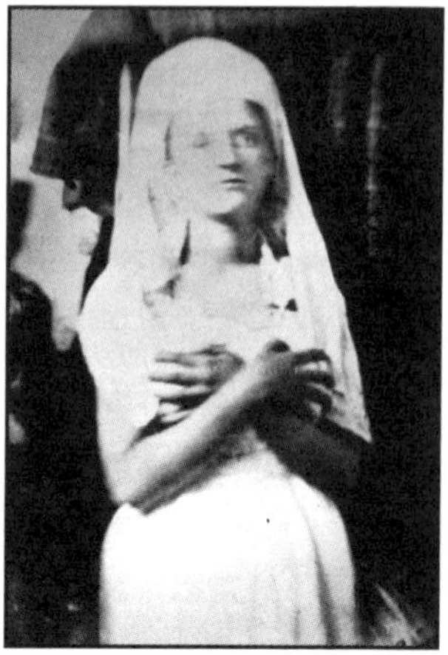

KATIE KING

At the end of the three years of experimentation, Katie King, in front of many photographic cameras, slowly dematerialized. She left for the scientists a materialized lock of her hair as final proof of the reality of her materialization. We are, therefore, stating facts that have already been demonstrated.

The encephalon is governed by the mind, yet the mind is not governed by the encephalon. The encephalon is the instrument of emotions and of the consciousness, yet the encephalon neither produces emotions nor consciousness. What is logic cannot be refuted by ignorance. Logic is logic. The people who affirm that the brain produces thought, emotion, and consciousness are ignorant, because they have not studied the Mental Body. So, we cannot, based on our ignorance, refute what is factual. It is necessary for the ignorant to study.

The twelve pairs of cranial nerves demonstrate to us the Hermetic principle that states, "As above, so below." If a zodiac with twelve constellations exists above, also here below, a zodiacal human being with his twelve pairs of cranial nerves exists. Each pair of nerves controls some region of the physical body. The twelve pairs of nerves control all the twelve parts of the zodiac human being. Such nerves are:

1. Olfactory nerves.
2. Optic nerves.
3. Oculomotor nerves.
4. Trochlear nerves.

5. Trigeminal nerves.
6. Abducens nerves.
7. Facial nerves.
8. Vestibulocochlear nerves.
9. Glossopharyngeal nerves.
10. Vagus nerves.
11. Spinal nerves.
12. Hypoglossal nerves.

These twelve pairs of nerves inform the mind of all that happens in the human zodiac. The office that collects that information is the brain and the office worker is the mind.

Thus, the organs of the senses of external perception collect the information that comes from the exterior world. Then, the information passes into the cerebral office where the office worker (the mind) analyzes and studies it. Unfortunately, the office worker has always a bad secretary who betrays him. That bad secretary is the "I," the myself, the ego.

For instance, we go to the movie-theater where we watch an erotic movie; there, the office worker within his cerebral suite collects all the perceptions. The office worker studies the movie; he contemplates it; he enjoys himself with it. Thereafter, the secretary, by his own whim, on the sly and in secrecy, plunders the erotic images and reproduces them in Nature's Mental Plane. This is how these images convert themselves into living effigies of the Mental Plane.

Later on, during our normal sleep, the mind, bottled up with the "I," fornicates with those mental effigies. This is why nocturnal pollutions occur.

The dreamer fornicates with the mental images that he, himself, created. The dreamer clairvoyantly sees those images. This is what is called unconscious clairvoyance.

Someone is jealous and supposes that a friend of his is having an affair with his spouse. Thus, his "jealous I," with those picture-fantasies created by himself, elaborates a drama in secrecy. Then, nocturnal dreams occur, and he sees horrible dramas where his spouse is committing adultery with his friend and many other terrible things. This is what is called unconscious clairvoyance.

If the clairvoyant is an oligophrenic, then he will vilely assassinate his friend. If he is neurasthenic, he then will insult, calumniate and finally assassinate him. If he is paranoid, he then will intellectually plan a technical and perfect assassination. If he is schizophrenic, he will violently break that friendship. If he is a sadomasochist, he will assassinate his spouse in the most horrible way. If he is a very cultured schizoid with a genotypic epileptic base, he then can receive a very intense emotional shock that will make him commit the crime of homicide and will fall afterwards into a global psychic state of collapse.

The majority of clairvoyants fall into the abyss of delinquency because of their lack of culture and intellectual discipline.

Let us suppose that a clairvoyant distrusts a friend because he assumes that he is a black magician. For that reason, he elaborates the most terrible forms within his unconsciousness; thereafter, these forms appear in his dreams. This is unconscious clairvoyance. This is why he can suffer a tremendous situational reaction that will take him into crime, calumny, public slander, defamation of character, assassination, etc.

All the unconscious clairvoyant perceptions enter the cerebellum. Thereafter, the cerebellum transfers such perceptions through the cell groups of the pons or breach, into the cerebrum. So, the unconscious perceptions become conscious when they enter the cerebrum.

The pons connects the midbrain with the medulla and with the two famous cerebral hemispheres.

In ancient times, the medulla oblongata constituted the whole brain, which could perfectly control all the cells of the human organism.

The medulla contains seven functional centers that govern sneezing, coughing, suction, mastication, deglutition, regurgitation, the functions of the salivary and gastric glands, and the closing of the eyelids.

The midbrain is also very interesting. Part of it joins the two cerebral hemispheres with the cerebellum and the pons or breach. Clairvoyant perceptions pass through the pons. All the centers that govern the human organism are located within the functional areas of the brain.

Many times a clairvoyant perception is recorded in a fixed way within one cerebral cell. This is similar to an image that is recorded on photographic film. In this case, the mind perceives at all hours such an unconscious clairvoyant image. Surgeons have resolved such a problem by extirpating the cell where the image is recorded.

A concrete case of unconscious clairvoyance and homicide was the assassination of the great Colombian politician Jorge Eliecer Gaitan. The investigations of the authorities had shown that the assassin was an active member of the school A.M.O.R.C. from San Jose, California. It was also stated that he was expelled from that school because they considered him a mentally unbalanced individual. Such a personage was an unconscious clairvoyant. He lit a pair of candles in front of his altar, in accordance with an A.M.O.R.C.-Rosicrucian ritual. Thus, in the mirror he saw two images, Simon Bolivar and Francisco de Paula Santander, who was Simon Bolivar's enemy.

Therefore, the assassin told himself, if Santander tried to kill me in my past reincarnation, now in my present existence I will take revenge on him and I will kill him. Thus, the 9th of April, the day of the events, he treacherously killed Jorge Elicer Gaitan when this politician was leaving the Government Palace of Bogota.

The experts on ballistics considered that the assassin, before such a homicide, had to have practiced a lot in the target range, since the three shots in the victim's back were well aimed, exact, and precise.

What happened afterwards was frightful. This Bogotanian assassin astonished the whole world. The excited crowds launched themselves to battle against the government. If, in the middle of such a situation, the cunning of a very fox-like liberal politician had not been present, the populace would have taken the Presidential Palace.

The former narrative is a concrete example of homicide and unconscious clairvoyance.

There is no doubt that the vision in the mirror was the secret source of such a crime. The political enemies of Gaitan made the rest. Possibly, they financed that crime; they bought the assassin, etc.

The secret source of this crime was unconscious clairvoyance. The unbalanced mind of the assassin created the images that were projected into the mirror. This is all.

Unconscious clairvoyance is the secret cause of one hundred percent of homicides.

Forensic psychiatry needs to expand itself a little more.

Many times, the perceptions from unconscious clairvoyance remain deposited within the unconscious depths of the human mind. Such perceptions convert themselves into secret temptation, which is the cause of many crimes. In the depths of every human being, many unconscious factors exist that often cause him to commit homicide. The secret sources of any crime are unconscious. Many saints had an unconsciousness filled with carnal passion, sadism, robbery, crime, violence, jealousy, hatred, resentments, etc., etc.

Such saints suffered horribly during their dream state. During their dreams, such saints fell into the most frightful crimes. Those saints were great evil doers within their unconsciousness. When they awakened from their dreams, they understood their frightful moral misery. Thus, this is why they were performing terrible penances and covering themselves with sackcloth.

Those who achieve making a moral defect into conscious consciousness will attain the total disintegration of such a defect.

When a human being disintegrates all of his defects, then his "I" is dissolved.

The truth comes into us when the "I" is dissolved. This is how we become perfect clairvoyants.

The truth is born from creative comprehension. The truth is non-temporal, eternal, and divine. The "I" cannot know the truth, because the "I" is just a bunch of memories. The "I" is of time. The "I" is born in time and dies in time. Death is just a subtraction of fractions. After finishing the mathematical operation (death), only the values remain. Later on, such values return into newborn physical bodies. Such values are the "I," the myself, the returning ego.

Therefore, the "I" is just illusion. Any crime, any felony, and any vice are the fatal outcome of the affirmation of the "I," of the myself. The origin of pain lies within the "I." The "I" is dissolved when we annihilate desire. Where the truth abides, the "I" cannot abide, because the truth and the "I" are incompatible.

The "I" is a transitory error of the Wheel of Samsara (the Wheel of Reincarnation and Karma). The "I" is the heresy of separatism.

The "I" is the origin of egotism, hatred, fornication, adultery, envy, anger, etc., etc. The "I" is the thirst of pleasures and the source of pride and vanity. Therefore, in order to incarnate the truth one needs to dissolve the "I." In order to attain internal peace, one needs to dissolve the "I," the myself. In order to acquire perfect clairvoyance and supreme illumination one needs to dissolve the "I."

The truth is the Internal Christ of every human being.

The "I" is the Satan that we carry inside.

Where the "I" is the truth cannot be.

Those who divide themselves into two "I's," one superior and another inferior, walk upon the path of error.

Those who affirm the existence of a divine "I" are making Satan godly.

A separated individual spirit does not exist. Only the Universal Spirit of Life exists.

Therefore, the immortal spark (Spirit) of every human being is the Being that is one with the Universal Spirit filled with supreme happiness.

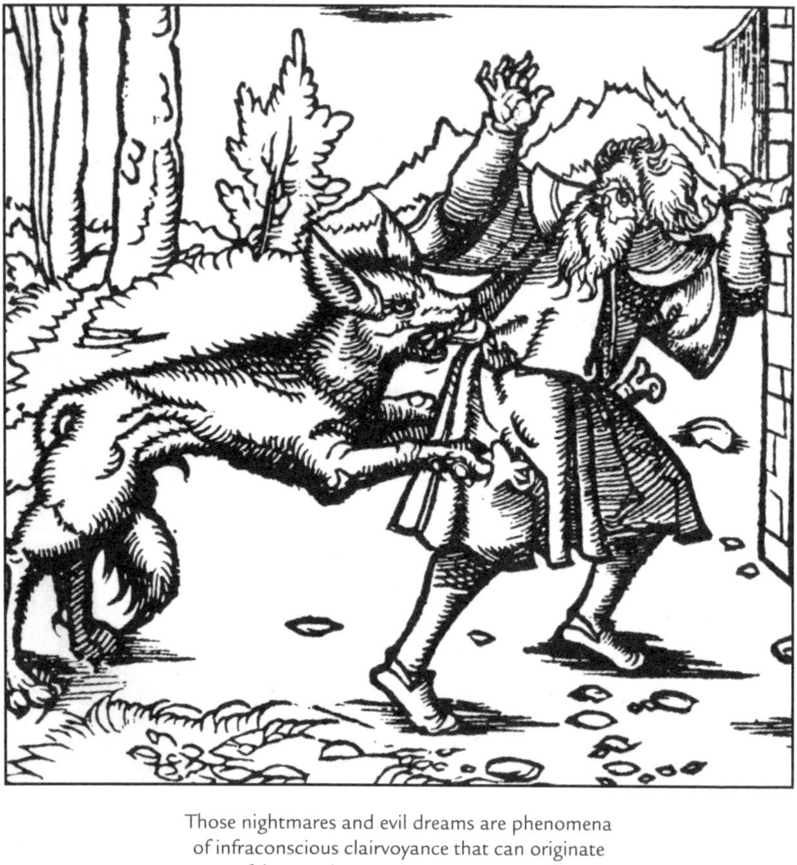

Those nightmares and evil dreams are phenomena of infraconscious clairvoyance that can originate false conclusions, resulting in crime.

Chapter 20
The Infraconsciousness

Infraconscious clairvoyance is commonly qualified and known by the name of nightmares. The dream's inebriation exists in the hypnotic crepuscular state.

The dream's inebriation has a longer duration than the hypnotic crepuscular state. The cerebral cortex intervenes notably in the dream's inebriation, not as a cause but as vehicle of the oneiric (dream) consciousness. The reflecting acts of the oneiric consciousness are the distinct varieties of somnambulism.

An intense action of the mesencephalon exists in the hypnotic crepuscular state. This intense action is not the cause but the effect of certain short circuits from psycho-infraconscious currents. These originate psychic effects and automatic acts that are sometimes criminal.

Subsequent lacunar amnesia with distinct degrees and tinges exists within the dream's inebration.

The sensation of amnesia caused by the definitively automatic action does not exist within the hypnotic crepuscular state. The common factor of both phenomena of psychic origin is the inhibition of the normal consciousness by the natural process of the dream.

Now, we mention an infraconscious clairvoyance case cited by Swartzer:

> "A woman from Pesth dreamed that a dog chased her and she was trying to reject it by stoning it. She, awakened by that nightmare, took her little girl who was sleeping by her side and threw her with violence, as if she was a stone, against the wall in order to scare the vicious dog."

Let us see another case of infraconscious clairvoyance cited by Kraft-Ebing:

> "In the middle of the night, a guardian heard from a house a scream of someone saying, "Help my children!" He entered the house and found a mother in her nightgown in an extremely excited and perturbed state. The whole room

> was in major disorder. Two children were crouched in a corner of the room. The woman was constantly screaming, "Where is my little boy? Did you take him? I think I threw him out through the window..."
>
> The unhappy woman had thrown her son outside onto the streets through the glass without opening the window. She had dreamed that her children were screaming at her and flames surrounded the house. Therefore, during her awakening mental confusion, she had cast her little boy through the window in order to protect him from the fire."
>
> (BUCKNILL, TUKE, AND LERB, 1862. PAGE 213).

We have found another case of infraconscious clairvoyance on page 203 in a book written by the doctors Diaz Padron and E. C. Henriquez:

> "Very late one night, a man who was alone in his apartment was dreaming that bandits were assaulting his home. Very strong knocks were heard from the door that was next to the stairs. The tenant awoke and rose holding a gun in his hand. He opened the door and shot the gun without seeing or aiming at anyone.
>
> "The bullet shot a young boy who carried an urgent telegram. When the homicidal one saw the deliverer of the telegram falling, he then became aware that he had just wounded an innocent person. In that moment, he completely awoke."

Those nightmares and evil dreams are phenomena of infraconscious clairvoyance that can originate false conclusions, resulting in crime.

When the clairvoyant is an neurasthenic occultist or esoterist, he can then become a premeditator and perfidious assassin.

An occultist student of a neurasthenic type was dreaming of a citizen. He was seeing with his infraconscious clairvoyance that such a citizen was tormenting him with witchcraft and black magic. A few days later, the neurasthenic insulted and threatened to death the perplexed and astonished citizen. This type of infraconscious vision with premeditation, calumny and perfidy is very common in some occultist and spiritualist students, etc.

The lack of mental appreciation of the infraconsciousness by esoterist or spiritualist clairvoyants is due to fanaticism and ignorance.

The mental disorder of ignorant fanatics is due to superstitious fear, to suggestion, and also to the lower aggressive instincts of their psycho-typic "I."

As the infraconsciousness exists within the human being, likewise it exists within Nature. The tenebrous memories of the whole history of the Earth and of its root races are deposited within the infraconsciousness of Nature. The antediluvian monsters live within the infraconsciousness of Nature. These are the spectres of the past, the nightmare phantoms.

The infraconscious clairvoyant only perceives the cavernous memories of the past and the tenebrous creations from the infraconscious lower depths of the human beings and beasts.

Fatality only exists within the infraconsciousness of nature.

Every human being has a double, an opposite, who lives within the infraconsciousness of Nature. In front of Buddha, we find his brother and enemy Devadatta, the King of hell. In front of Anael, the Angel of Love, we find Lilith, the antithesis of love.

An infraconscious clairvoyant may see the double of someone and thereafter deduce erroneous conclusions whose final outcome is calumny, homicide, etc., etc.

The infraconsciousness is the tenebrous remnant from a remote past. The sadomasochist is the sexual pervert that can assassinate his spouse just for pure sexual pleasure. This sexual perversion is infraconscious. The infraconscious values of the psychological "I" constitute the lowest animal depths of the human being.

The tyrannical, obsessive, sexual perversion of the sadomasochist is the concrete manifestation of his infraconscious values.

When this genre of infraconscious values flourishes in his mind, the human being falls into crimes like homosexuality, stupor, force, violence, corruption of minors, etc. Sometimes, such a sexual pervert becomes a mystic, an ignoramus, a sanctimonious one, etc.

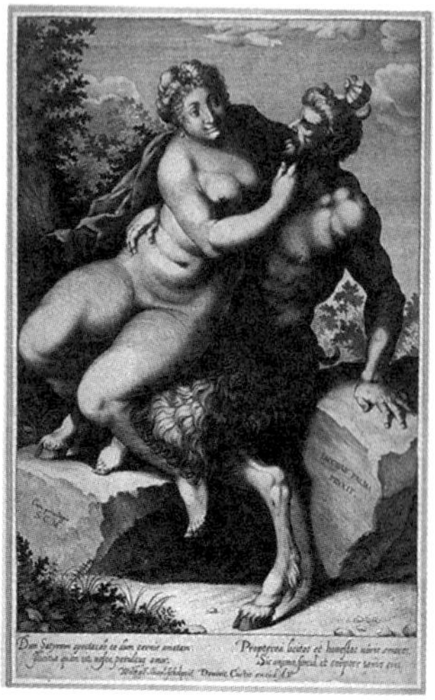

We knew the case of a mystical sexual pervert who used to give away coins to six and seven year old girls "for their candies." This is how he was cultivating them while they were aging a little. Afterwards, he was sexually seducing them, and finally in order to avoid conflicts and problems, he engaged them with other men. Nonetheless, such a satyr was a mystic spiritualist who filled with sweetness was always smiling. He was a hierarch from a Spiritualist Society.

Many times, the sexual perversion of the infraconsciousness places its satyrs in the arena of compulsive psychoneurosis that causes them to commit the most terrible crimes registered by the police news chronicles.

Sexual infraconscious perversion has two very well defined poles: the brain and sexuality. Thieves are positive; prostitutes are negative. These are the two poles of the human infraconsciousness. Observe the intimate psychic affinity that exists between prostitutes and thieves.

These two poles of the human infraconsciousness live in an eternal struggle within each individual. We see clearly in the example of the spiritualist satyr cited in this present chapter the struggle of the infraconsciousness.

The satyr's brain cultivates the girls with coins for their candies and waits a little while for their aging. Then, the satyr's sexuality possesses and consummates the crime of seduction. The satyr's brain projects and plans; afterwards, he engages the girls with other men in order to avoid conflicts. Behold here the struggle between brain and sexuality.

Many times the infraconsciousness betrays a virtuous spouse and carries her towards adultery. Many prostitutes who in their past were magnificent spouses live in brothels. When the sexual perversion of these harlots polarizes itself in their brain, drained by pleasure, then they commit terrible crimes that take them to jail.

These incarcerated, unhappy women feel themselves victims of human injustice; they consider themselves innocent. Indeed, those women are victims of an energy that they ignore. No one has cured such unhappy ones, not a single psychiatrist has taught them how to use and drive their sexual energy. They do not know the great mysteries of sex.

They are victims of a society that, after perverting them, despises and miserably humiliates them.

Society corrupts these unhappy women, daughters of pain, in order to confine them within horrible panoptics and in jails where they only end up perverting themselves still more.

The infraconsciousness cannot be confined within jails.

The delinquent does not reform himself in jails. The jail system has become a complete failure. Inside jails, the delinquents multiply their hatred and rancor against society.

The sexual problems in jails, the homosexuality and all kinds of filthy vices against nature, are showing us until satiation that the infraconsciousness cannot be confined within jails.

The biggest sin is ignorance.

Only with a wise pedagogic psychotherapy can the reform of delinquents be achieved. The corrective pedagogic treatment within jails can transform them into true reformatory schools. Jails should not exist. Only reformatory schools, etc. should exist. In these schools, the delinquents can be cured with Pedagogic Psychotherapy.

Convicts must be treated with infinite love and mercy.

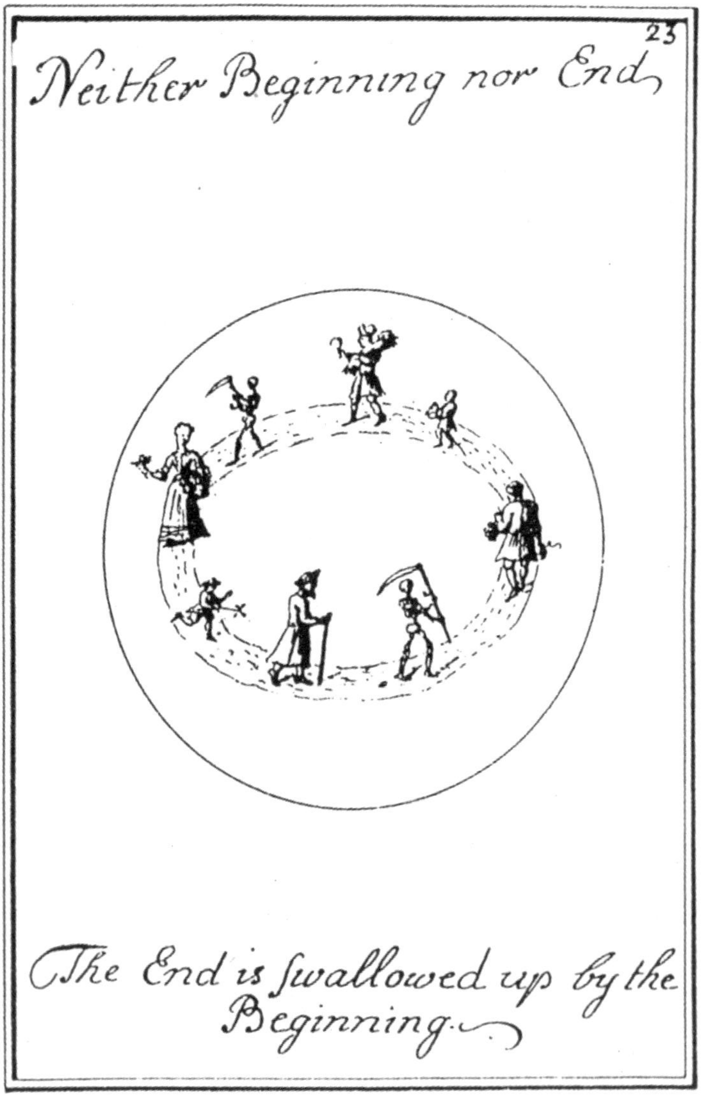
23
Neither Beginning nor End
The End is swallowed up by the Beginning.

Everything that is sown within the subconsciousness flourishes in the mind throughout time.

Chapter 21

The Subconsciousness

When a criminal is psychogenically analyzed, the subconscious factors have to be taken into account.

These types of factors are reduced into three, namely: **Genotype** (inheritance), **Phenotype** (education), **Paratype** (circumstances). The upright social conduct of any individual is the outcome of the perfect equilibrium among these three factors.

When a disequilibrium among these three factors exists, then the outcome is crime. These three factors can be positive or negative.

They are positive when they manifest themselves as upright thoughts, upright feelings, and upright actions.

They are negative when they manifest themselves as criminal thoughts, criminal feelings, and criminal actions.

Let us study these three factors separately.

Inheritance is the vehicle of Karma, Nemesis or Law of Destiny. Here, we are not asking you to believe, you may not believe in it. However, what we need is to analyze and to profoundly delve into the distinct inner-depths of the mind.

Concerning beliefs, to say, "I believe or I do not believe," is proper for ignorant people. We are mathematicians in our scientific investigations and very demanding in our analysis and our expression.

Death is a subtraction operation. When such an arithmetic operation is finished, only the values remain. These values are what continue.

These values constitute the psychological "I," the myself, the ego, that reincarnates in order to satisfy its frustrated desires and in order to continue existing though a new personality.

The "I" is a bunch of memories, passions, desires, hatreds, violence, lust, greed, etc., etc. The "I" constitutes such values. Such energetic values are anterior to the seminal germinal cell.

If we investigate all the intra-atomic and inter-atomic states of the seminal germinal cell, we only find electricity and magnetism.

We are not settling dogmas. Let us perform the test. Let us take the seminal germinal cell into an atomic physics laboratory. Thus, if we fraction asunder the atom of the seminal germinal cell, we will then liberate energy, because according to atomic physics, any atom is an exponent of energies.

If a scientific clairvoyant would analyze those liberated energies of the atom from the seminal germinal cell, he then will find the reincarnating ego (the values).

Existence begins with the cell that is elaborated within the man's testicles and prostate. This cell (sperm) is decapitated when entering within the maternal ovum.

The factors of inheritance are deposited in the genes. The word *gene* comes from the same Greek root which originates the words *genesis, generation, genre,* etc.

The genes are within small bar forms that are named chromosomes. The paternal and maternal inheritance is in within the genes.

Inheritance is the vehicle of the cruel Nemesis of life.

Inheritance is the outcome of Karma (the Law of Action and Consequence, Nemesis).

> *For with what measure ye mete, it shall be measured to you again.*
>
> - MATTHEW: 7: 2.

Such as the action is, such is how the consequence will be. This is the law.

We carry the outcome of our past evil deeds within our inheritance. Axiomatically speaking, we state the following: evil actions are the *causa causorum* of inheritance.

This axiom is comprehensible when we understand the Law of Reincarnation and of Nemesis (Karma).

The values of a man who was an artist will reincarnate in a family of artists who will provide the necessary genetic inheritance for him.

A sum of mystic values will reincarnate among compassionate people.

The values of a libertine person will reincarnate among libertine people. The values of an assassin will reincarnate among assassins and thieves.

It has happened many times, cases of saints reincarnating among bandits and vice versa. When this happens, it is the law of destiny adjusting accounts.

We carry within our subconsciousness all of that inheritance. The factors of our inheritance betray us many times.

Now, let us analyze **education**. This second factor of the subconsciousness is very important. Education begins at home. The child learns more through example than from precept.

The child witnesses in modern homes the adultery of his parents.

The child is an eyewitness of the anger, greed, and lust of those who gave him life.

The child sees with astonishment in his home the revolver or the rifle of his father and the magazines or the tales of assassins and thieves, etc.

The child goes to the movies where he enjoys watching scenarios of detectives against thieves who assault people in the roads or who assault banks. When the night of Christmas or any other holiday arrives, the child receives cannon, revolver and pistol toys. So, the child can then play as a bandit or a thief who assaults people in the roads, etc.

All of these remain stored within the subconsciousness of the child.

The child's parents themselves are the ones who poison him little by little with the fatal venom of delinquency.

Time passes away, the child grows, and the ideas of crime that were deposited within his subconsciousness develop, evolve, and progress. This subconsciously occurs even when the child's vital conscious part ignores everything that happens within the profound regions of his subconsciousness. Any given day the fruit (ideas of crime) ripens and the harvest is crime.

Everything that is sown within the subconsciousness flourishes in the mind throughout time.

The situational reaction of a homicidal one who never wanted to kill is the fatal outcome of all of that which he learned when he was a child.

The new gangster, the street-smart thief, the new housebreaker who was before a good citizen, is the outcome of a false education.

Pornographic, erotic novels and movies engender prostitution, seduction and abduction with force and violence, etc., etc.

The pornographic movie actors and writers are teaching perversities onto the subconsciousness of children and adults. Therefore, the time to fight against the moral corruption from the prostitutes of intelligence has arrived.

The child learns in school bloody histories of slyness, maliciousness, distrust, etc., etc., that are recorded within the subconsciousness. With all of this recorded within the subconsciousness, the fatal outcome is crime.

Now, let us study **circumstances**, certain critical circumstances that irritate the subconsciousness and provoke criminal reactions.

Objective circumstances combine themselves with similar subconscious circumstances within the subconsciousness in order to provoke crime.

Objective and subjective images combine themselves in order to provoke crime. Example: an unemployed man, hungry and miserable, remembers having seen, in his infancy, his father in the same crisis. Then, he remembers that his father, in order to solve the problem, assaulted a person in the streets and robbed him. Then he remembers the good food that was served at the table of his home after the robbery, etc.

Therefore, the critical circumstance of the unemployed man together with the circumstance of his subconscious remembrance combine and provoke the crime.

The three factors Genotype, Phenotype, and Paratype are the Psychogenesis of every criminal act.

Crime can be extirpated from its more intimate roots only with an integral culture.

Crime can be extirpated from the mind only with an integral culture.

The subconscious clairvoyant only perceives the history of the human race throughout the centuries. The memories of all our past reincarnations live within our subconsciousness. Many times a subconscious clairvoyant falls into crime when seeing a remembrance. For example, it can happen that a subconscious clairvoyant may clairvoyantly see his loyal spouse committing adultery. The clairvoyant is sure of his vision; he knows the word hallucination has been invented by ignoramuses in order to disguise their own ignorance. He knows that the vision exists.

If the clairvoyant is a non-cultured individual without intellectual discipline of any kind, then he will react in accordance to his bio-psychological "I."

If he is a neurasthenic clairvoyant he will treacherously assassinate his spouse after having vilely slandered her as an adulterer.

The paranoid clairvoyant will intellectually project a very intelligent crime.

The epileptic type of clairvoyant will momentarily react with an explosive outburst of brutal anger. Then, after having broken through his explosive anger, his phenotypic superstructure of personal control, created by his social habits and his education, he will madly drag himself to assassinate his virtuous and loyal spouse.

The oligophrenic clairvoyant would commit a filthy and horrifying crime. This is how he would assassinate his loyal spouse.

The schizophrenic clairvoyant would abandon her immediately.

The sadomasochist clairvoyant would assassinate her during the very sexual act or after it.

These are the dangers of subconscious clairvoyance. The clairvoyant does not doubt his vision. He thinks that his vision is not a hallucination.

If the subconscious clairvoyant does not study Psychiatry, Theosophy, Psychology, Rosicrucianism, etc., etc., he can then fall into the most horrifying crimes. The loyal spouse of our example could have been an adulterer in her past reincarnation. Therefore, the clairvoyant without discipline and intellectual culture will ignore what the past and the subconsciousness are. The outcome of his ignorance and his lack of culture, is crime, public slander, etc., etc.

In many spiritualistic schools, the subconscious clairvoyants may skin their neighbors alive. They calumniate the innocent; they accuse them of witchcraft, sorcery, black magic, adultery, robbery, extortion, etc. Nobody escapes them; they slander everyone.

It is peculiar to see those subconscious clairvoyants as proud ignoramuses who boast of being wise. They foretell infamies. They torment their neighbors by accusing good citizens. They base their actions on their subconscious clairvoyance. They clairvoyantly see people in the old past of their ancient lives, committing errors that in their present life they are incapable of committing.

The penal code should also punish the calumniator clairvoyants.

Constantly, we hear those subconscious calumniator clairvoyants utter phrases such as the following: "A fellow is a Black Magician and he is putting a spell on me," or "The lady 'X' is committing adultery with the gentleman 'Y.'"

They affirm it, even when the slandered woman may be a saint. Those clairvoyant ignoramuses lack respect for others.

Nevertheless, we cannot blame their clairvoyance. Indeed, the sixth sense is as natural and normal as the eyes, the ears, the olfactory sense, the mouth, and the sense of touch.

The clairvoyant is not to blame for those errors. The cause of all of those errors is the lack of intellectual culture and the lack of respect towards our neighbor.

The memories of all of those errors that we committed in our past reincarnations live within our subconsciousness. The clairvoyant without intellectual culture sees all of those errors from the past, then he gets confused and the outcome is calumny against just and honorable people.

The cultured clairvoyant, the intellectual clairvoyant, who has studied Psychiatry, Theosophy, Psychology, Rosicrucianism, etc., etc., does not fall into such errors, because he has intellectual discipline. The cultured, educated, respectful and intellectually disciplined clairvoyant, enjoys the illuminated intellection, he knows how to read in the subconsciousness of nature with complete cognizance.

The cultured, educated, respectful, and intellectually disciplined clairvoyant is capable of retrospectively studying the whole history of the Earth and its Root Races. He is an illuminated clairvoyant.

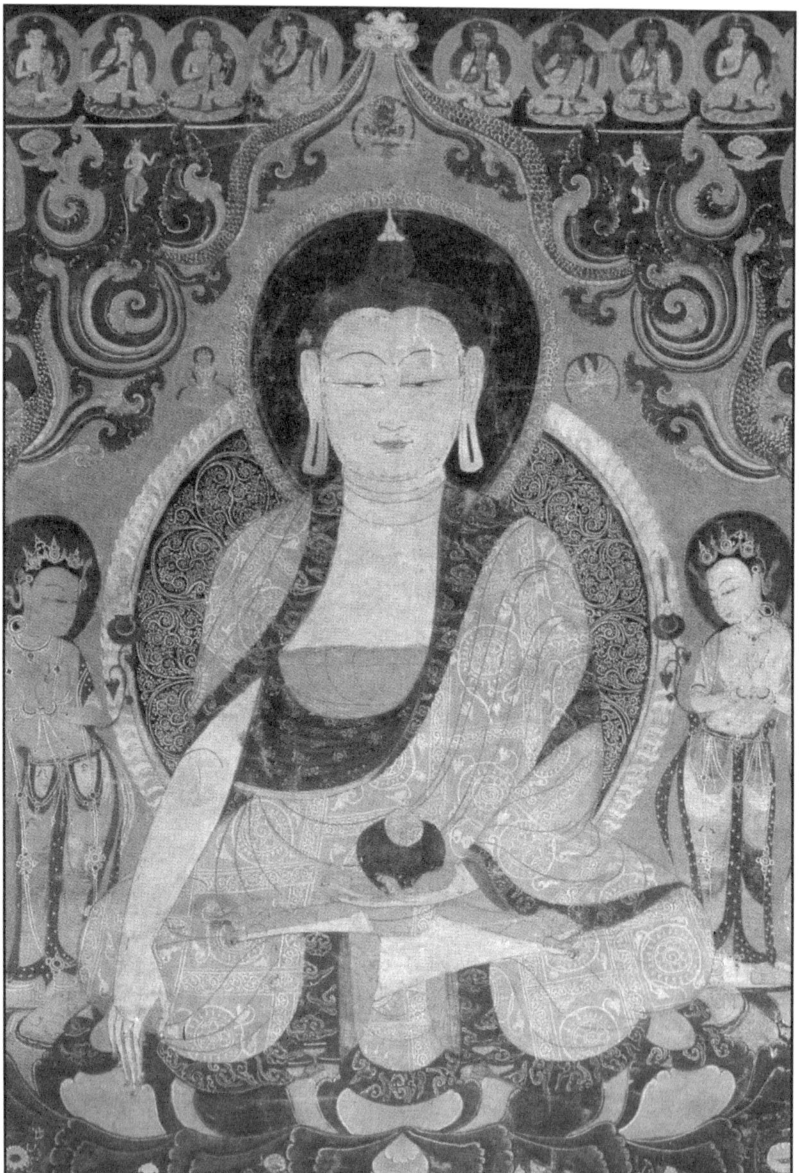

The Buddha Shakyamuni

The triple way of science, philosophy, and revolutionary cosmic mysticism conduces us into the ineffable regions of the great Light.

Chapter 22

The Supraconsciousness

The most elevated type of clairvoyance that exists in the universe is the **supraconsciousness**. All the avatars or messengers from the superior worlds have been supraconscious clairvoyants. Hermes Trismegistus, Rama, Krishna, Buddha, Jesus Christ, etc., are supraconscious beings, messengers of the superior worlds, initiators of new eras of historic evolution.

Imagination, Inspiration, and Intuition are the three obligatory steps of the Initiation. We are going to examine each one of these three steps separately.

Let us begin with Imagination.

Imagination

For the wise, to imagine is to see. Imagination is the translucence of the soul.

What is important is to learn to concentrate thought on one thing only.

Whosoever learns to think on only one thing creates marvels and prodigies.

The disciple who wants to reach Imaginative Knowledge must learn to concentrate himself and know how to profoundly meditate.

The best exercise in order to attain Imaginative Knowledge is the following:

While seated in front of a plant, we concentrate on it until we forget everything that is not related with it. Then, by closing the eyes, we become drowsy and keep in our imagination the form, figure, structure, perfume and color of the plant.

The disciple must provoke drowsiness during these practices.

The disciple, while in drowsiness, will profoundly meditate on the internal constitution of the plant.

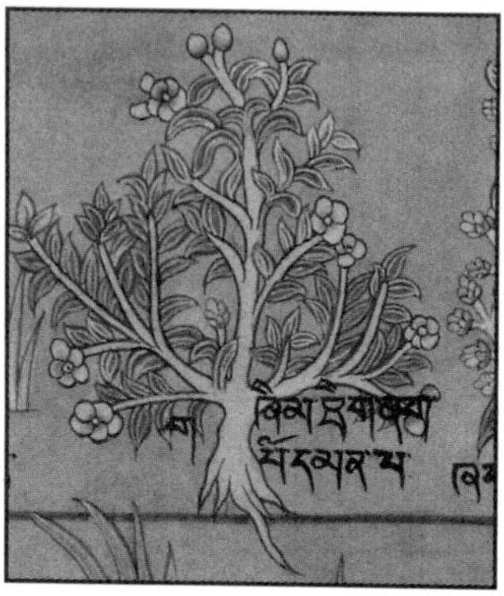

The disciple will imagine the living cells of the plant. Each cell possesses protoplasm, membrane and nucleus. The protoplasm is a viscose, elastic, and transparent substance, similar to the egg white (albuminoid matter). The disciple, while in drowsiness, must reflect upon the four fundamental elements in the protoplasm of the cell of the plant. These four elements are carbon, oxygen, hydrogen and nitrogen.

The membrane is a marvelous substance without color, a substance within which the water becomes totally insoluble. This substance is the well-known cellulose.

The disciple, while concentrated, will imagine the nucleus of the cell as a small corpuscle where the great universal life palpitates. The nuclear filament is within the nucleus, as well as the nuclear juice and the nucleolus which are all covered by the nuclear membrane. The nucleoli are infinitesimal corpuscles filled with brightness and beauty. These are residual products of the incessant reactions of the plant organism.

The disciple, while well-concentrated, must imagine with complete logical precision all of those mineral substances and organic combinations that are harmoniously unfolding within the cellular protoplasm of the plant. Let us think on the grains of starch and on the portentous chlorophyll, without which it is impossible to reach the perfect organic synthesis. The chlorophyll is presented in granulated form (chloro-leucite) as a very beautiful yellow color (xanthophyll) that becomes that precious green color of the plant while under the solar rays.

Every plant is a perfect cellular community with incalculable perfections. The student must meditate on the perfection of the plant and on all of its scientific processes. He must be filled with a mystic attitude and enchanted with so much beauty.

The mystic is in rapture when remembering all of the phenomena of nutrition, relation, and reproduction of each cell of the plant.

Let us see the chalice of the flower. Here are its sexual organs; here is the pollen, the masculine reproductive element; here is the pistil or gynoecium, a very precious feminine organ with its ovary, stylus, and stigma.

The ovary is a sack full of marvelous ovums. The stamen can occupy different positions in relation with the pistil, for instance, insertion beneath the ovary, insertion around the ovary, or above it.

Fecundation is verified with the function of the feminine germs and masculine gametes. After exiting the anther, the pollen, the masculine gamete, reaches the ovary of the plant where the ovum, the feminine gamete, is waiting with anxiety.

The seed is the precious and enchanted ovum that after being fecundated is transformed and grows.

Now the student should remember the step on which he is meditating. A sprout will emerge as a delicate bud; imagine it growing slowly, until seeing it with your imagination spreading branches, leaves, and flowers. Remember that everything that is born must die. Imagine the plant's process of dying. Its flowers wither; its leaves dry and the wind blows them away. Finally, only a few twigs remain.

This process of birth and death is marvelous. By meditating on the whole process of the birth and death of a plant, by meditating on its marvelous life, if the concentration is perfect and a profound level of drowsiness is achieved, then the chakras of the Astral Body will spin, develop, and unfold.

Meditation must be correct. The mind must be exact. Logical thought and exact concept is needed for the purpose of developing the internal senses absolutely perfectly.

Every incoherence, every lack of logical and moral equilibrium obstructs and damages the evolution and progress of the chakras, disks, or lotus flowers of the Astral Body.

The student needs a lot of patience, because any act of impatience takes him into failure.

The student needs a lot of patience, willpower, tenacity, and absolutely conscious faith.

On any given day, within dreams or while in meditation, a distant picture, a landscape of nature, a feature, etc. emerges. This is a sign that the student is progressing.

The student elevates himself little by little into Imaginative Knowledge. The student is unveiling the veil of Isis little by little.

On any given day, the plant on which he was meditating disappears. Then, a beautiful child who replaces the plant is seen. That child is the elemental of the plant, the soul of the plant.

Later, during a dream, he awakens his consciousness, then he can say, "I am in my Astral Body." The consciousness awakens little by little. In this way, the moment in which the disciple will acquire Continuous Consciousness arrives.

When the student enjoys Continuous Consciousness, he no longer dreams; he can no longer dream, because his consciousness is awakened. Then, even when the physical body is sleeping, he moves himself consciously in the superior worlds.

Exact meditation awakens the internal senses and performs a complete transformation of the internal bodies.

Whosoever awakens consciousness has reached Imaginative Knowledge. This one moves in the world of symbolic images.

The symbols that the student saw while he was dreaming he now sees without dreaming, as before he was seeing them with a sleeping consciousness. Now he moves himself among them with an awakened consciousness even when his physical body is profoundly asleep.

When the student reaches Imaginative Knowledge, he sees the symbols but he does not understand them. He comprehends that all of nature is a living scripture that he does not know. The student needs to elevate himself into Inspired Knowledge in order to interpret the sacred symbols of Great Nature.

Let us now study Inspiration.

Inspiration

Inspired Knowledge grants us the power of interpreting the symbols of Great Nature. The interpretation of symbols is very delicate. Many clairvoyants have become homicidal or have fallen into the crime of public slander because of not knowing how to interpret symbols.

Symbols must be analyzed coldly without superstition, maliciousness, mistrust, pride, vanity, fanaticism, prejudgment, preconceptions, hatred, envy, greed, jealousy, etc. All defects belong to the "I", to the myself, to the reincarnating ego.

When the "I" interferes by translating and interpreting symbols, then it alters the meaning of this secret scripture, and the clairvoyant falls into a crime that can conduct him to jail.

Interpretation must be tremendously analytical, highly scientific, and essentially mystical. There is a need to learn how to see and how to interpret in the absence of the "I," of the myself.

It seems very strange to many mystics that we the brothers and sisters of the International Gnostic Movement speak of divine clairvoyance with the penal code in hand. Those that think in this way consider spirituality as something that has nothing to do with our relationship to daily life. These people act wrongly and they are mistaken. They ignore what each soul is in the superior worlds: the exact outcome of daily life that every one of us lives in this valley of tears.

If our words, thoughts, and actions are not just, then the outcome appears in the internal worlds and the Law falls upon us.

The Law is the Law; to be ignorant of the Law does not mean the exclusion of its fulfillment. The worst sin is ignorance.

Therefore, to teach unto the one who does not know is a work of mercy. The whole tremendous responsibility of the Law falls upon the clairvoyant.

There is a need to interpret symbols of the great Nature in the absolute absence of the "I."

Nonetheless, self-criticism must be multiplied, because when the "I" of the clairvoyant believes he knows a lot, then he feels himself infallible, omniscient, wise and even supposes that he sees and interprets with the absence of the "I." These types of clairvoyants fortify the "I" so much that they end up converting themselves into terribly perverse demons. When a clairvoyant of this type sees his inner God, he interprets the vision in accordance with his tenebrous criteria and exclaims, "I am doing well."

Therefore, it is necessary to know how to interpret based on the Law of Philosophical Analogies, the Law of Correspondences and the numerical Kabbalah.

We recommend *The Mystical Qabbalah* by Dion Fortune and my book *Tarot and Kabbalah*. These books are essential; study them.

The one who has hatred, resentment, jealousy, envy, pride, etc. does not achieve elevation of himself to the second step called Inspired Knowledge.

When we elevate ourselves to Inspired Knowledge, we understand and comprehend that the accidental accumulation of objects does not exist.

Indeed, all phenomena of nature and all objects are found intimately and organically joined together, internally dependent upon each other and mutually conditioning each other.

Indeed, no phenomena of nature can be integrally comprehended if we consider it isolated.

Everything is in incessant movement. Everything changes; nothing is quiet.

In every object, the internal struggle exists. An object is positive and negative at the same time. Quantitative transforms itself into qualitative. Evolution is a process of the complication of energy.

Inspired Knowledge permits us to know the inner relationship between everything that is, has been, and will be.

Matter is nothing but condensed energy. The infinite modifications of energy are absolutely unknown, as much for the historic materialism as for the dialectic materialism.

Energy is equal to mass by the velocity of the light to the square. We, the Gnostics, separate ourselves from the antithetical struggle that exists between Metaphysics and Dialectic Materialism. These are the two antitheses of ignorance, the two antitheses of error.

We go in a distinct way. We are Gnostics. We consider life an integral whole.

The object is a point in space that serves as a vehicle to a determined sum of values.

Inspired Knowledge allows us to study the intimate existing relationships among all forms and values of this great Nature.

Dialectic Materialism does not know the values; it only studies the object. Metaphysics neither knows the values nor the object.

We, the Gnostics, separate ourselves from the two antitheses of ignorance, and we integrally study the human being and the Great Nature.

Life is every determined and determinant energy. Life is object and subject at the same time.

The disciple who wants to reach Inspired Knowledge must concentrate profoundly on classical music. *The Magic Flute* of Mozart reminds us of an Egyptian Initiation. The Nine Symphonies of Beethoven and many other great classical compositions elevate us to the superior worlds.

The disciple, profoundly concentrated in the music, must imbibe himself within it as the bee does within the honey, which is the product of his whole labor.

When the disciple has already reached Inspired Knowledge, he must then prepare himself for Intuitive Knowledge.

Let us now study Intuitive Knowledge.

Intuition

The world of intuition is the world of mathematics. The student that wants to elevate himself to the world of intuition must be a mathematician or at least must have notions of arithmetic.

Mathematical formulas grant us Intuitive Knowledge.

The student must concentrate himself on a mathematical formula and profoundly meditate on it. Afterwards, he must empty the mind and make it completely blank, then simply wait for the Inner Being to teach the contained concept which is enclosed in the mathematical formula.

For example: before Kepler publicly announced his famous principle that, "The square of the period of revolution of a planet varies directly as the distance from the sun cubed," that formula already existed; it was contained in the solar system, even when the wise did not know it.

The student can mentally concentrate himself on that formula. He must empty his mind, become drowsy. With his mind completely blank he must wait for his own inner Being to reveal to him all of the marvelous secrets which are contained in the formula of Kepler.

The formula of Newton concerning universal gravity can also serve us in order to exercise ourselves in the Initiation. This formula is the following: "The force between two objects varies directly with each of the masses and inversely with the square of the distance between them."

If the student practices with tenacity and supreme patience, his own inner Being will teach or instruct him in the Great Work. Then he will study at the feet of the Master and he will elevate himself to Intuitive Knowledge.

Imagination, Inspiration, and Intuition are obligatory steps of the Initiation. Whosoever has raised these three steps of direct knowledge has reached supraconsciousness.

In the world of Intuition, we find only omniscience. The world of intuition is the world of the Being; it is the world of the Intimate.

In this world, the "I," the myself, the ego, cannot enter.

The world of Intuition is the Universal Spirit of life.

The world of Imaginative Knowledge is a world of symbolic images.

Inspiration grants us the power of interpreting symbols.

In the world of Intuition, we see the great cosmic theater and we are the spectators. We attend the great drama of life.

In the world of Intuition, the whole drama, which is represented in cosmic scenes, is reduced to terrible arithmetical operations. This is the amphitheater of cosmic science.

From that region of mathematics, we see that physical masses exist that are above and below all of the limits of external sensorial perceptions. Those masses are invisible. We can perceive them only with clairvoyance.

Matter is condensed energy. When its vibration is very slow, its mass is beneath the limits of external sensorial perceptions. When its vibratory movement is very fast, then the mass is above the limits of external sensorial perceptions.

With the telescope, we can only see worlds whose degree of vibration is active within the limits of external sensorial perceptions.

Above and below the limits of external sensorial perceptions, worlds, solar systems, and constellations populated by many types of living beings exist.

The so-called matter is only energy that condenses into infinite masses.

The senses of external perception can only reach a fraction of what is perceivable.

In this day and age, Dialectic Materialism and Metaphysics are absolutely antiquated.

We, the brothers and sisters of the Gnostic movement, go in a distinct way.

It is urgent that scientists study the *Treatise of Occult Science* by Dr. Rudolf Steiner, the great Hungarian medic, born in 1861, friend and disciple of Nietzsche and Ernest Hegel. Dr. Rudolf Steiner is the founder of the Anthroposophic Society.

It is indispensable that those who are lovers of science investigate in depth the whole portentous oriental wisdom poured as a river of gold in the immortal pages of *The Secret Doctrine.* This work consists of six volumes and is a monument of the archaic wisdom.

The great master Helena Petrovna Blavatsky is the genius author of this precious treasury of ancient wisdom.

Those who reach the supraconsciousness convert themselves into true illuminated clairvoyants. No authentic clairvoyant boasts about his faculties.

No legitimate clairvoyant says that he is a clairvoyant.

When a true clairvoyant sees something important, he gives his concepts in a very cultured way and with supreme respect for others. He never says, "I am seeing." He always says, "We recognize, we have learned." This is how all of those that have reached the ineffable summits of supraconsciousness distinguish themselves by their gentility, humility, and modesty.

Powerful anthropological, cultural, intellectual, and universal Gnostic schools exist, AGLA. Study in them the Gnostic Doctrine.

You should read *Kundalini Yoga* by Sivananda. Meditate on the blessed White Lodge. Inquire within the Gnostic Treasuries.

Those who reach the heights of supraconsciousness enter into the amphitheater of cosmic science.

The triple way of science, philosophy, and revolutionary cosmic mysticism conduces us into the ineffable regions of the great Light.

Gnosis is highly scientific, highly philosophical, and transcendentally mystical.

Chapter 23

The Krishnamurti Case

A great conflict occurred inside the Theosophical Society during those times when Annie Besant was occupying the presidency of this marvelous organization, whose founder was the Great Initiate Helena Petrovna Blavatsky.

The problem that presented itself was the Krishnamurti case.

Lady Besant lifted her finger aloft in order to asseverate to the four winds that the Hindu boy Krishnamurti was the living reincarnation of Jesus Christ.

The great clairvoyant Leadbeater and other eminent Theosophists totally agreed with Lady Besant. All of them were asserting that the Hindustani boy was Jesus Christ newly reincarnated.

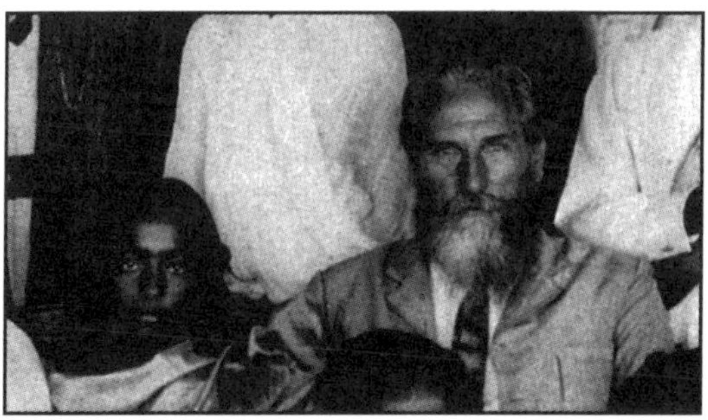

THE YOUNG KRISHNAMURTI WITH C. LEADBEATER

We still remember that foundation of that order named "The Star of the East" whose unique purpose was to welcome the Messiah. Later on, Krishnamurti himself dissolved it.

A division occurred within the bosom of the Theosophical Society in that epoch.

Some of them were asserting that Krishnamurti was the Messiah. Others did not accept such a concept; thus, they withdrew from the Theosophical Society.

The powerful illuminated clairvoyant, eminent intellectual, founder of the Anthroposophic Society, Dr. Rudolf Steiner, appears among those who withdrew.

The work of Rudolf Steiner is grandiose. His books are wells of profound wisdom.

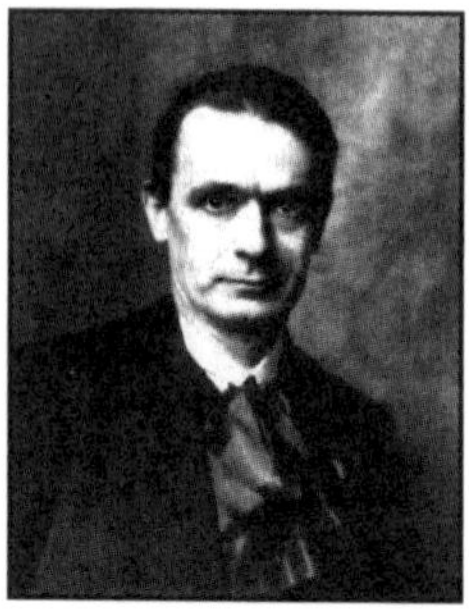

DR. RUDOLF STEINER

The Spaniard group Marco Aurelio also withdrew from the Theosophical Society.

The incision that occurred within the bosom of that famous Theosophical Society was a true tragedy.

We need to analyze the Krishnamurti case.

While some Theosophists were convinced that Krishnamurti was the reincarnation of Jesus Christ, others stated that he was just an ignorant boy. They stated that the only thing he knew was how to drive an automobile and play tennis, etc.

So, what was the matter? Why did they not agree?

What is most intriguing is that the greatest clairvoyants from the Theosophical Society were divided into two opposite bands.

Absolutely logical questions emerge: why did the clairvoyants divide among themselves?

These clairvoyants saw the internal Being of the Hindu boy. Why then did they not agree? Is it perhaps because some clairvoyants see in one way and other clairvoyants in another distinct way? Is it possible that the clairvoyants contradict among themselves? If the clairvoyants saw the inner Being of Jiddu Krishnamurti, what was the motivation for their disagreement?

When a thousand people see with their physical sight an object, they say: "This is a table, a chair, a rock, etc., etc." When they see a person they say: "This is a man or a woman or a child, etc." Then, what is going on with clairvoyance? What is the motive in this concrete case of this Hindu boy in which the clairvoyants could not agree in their concepts? There is no doubt that Krishnamurti was a true puzzle for the Theosophical Society.

The most critical thing was to see those clairvoyants fighting among themselves.

This is something that confuses the minds of those that until now are starting these studies.

Krishnamurti fell into skepticism. He remained skeptical for many years; yet, he finally reacted and started his mission.

All of us, the endoteric Gnostic Brethren, proposed ourselves to investigate the Krishnamurti case within the superior worlds.

After many patient works, we arrived at the following conclusions:

First: Every human being is a trio of body, Soul, and Spirit.

Second: When the Spirit defeats matter, he becomes a Buddha.

Third: When the Soul purifies and sanctifies itself, then it is called a bodhisattva.

Fourth: The Spirit of Krishnamurti is a Buddha.

Fifth: The Soul of Krishnamurti is a bodhisattva.

Many Buddhas exist in Asia who have not incarnated the Christ yet.

A ray that unites us to the Absolute exists within every human being.

That ray is our Resplendent Dragon of Wisdom, the Internal Christ, the Sephirotic Crown.

The Buddhas who have not incarnated the internal Christ, have not Christified themselves yet.

Krishnamurti's Buddha has already incarnated his Resplendent Dragon of Wisdom, his particular Ray, his own Internal Christ.

When Lady Besant, Leadbeater, and other Theosophists studied the Krishnamurti case, they became astonished with the splendid light of that Christified Buddha. However, since they did not know the Christic Esotericism, they completely believed that Krishnamurti was the reincarnation of Jesus Christ.

The mistake was not in their clairvoyance; the mistake was in their lack of intellectual culture. They only knew about the Theosophical Septenary. They only knew about the body, Soul, and Spirit. Yet, they ignored that beyond these three aspects (body, Soul, and Spirit) every human being has a Ray (the Internal Christ) that unites us to the Absolute.

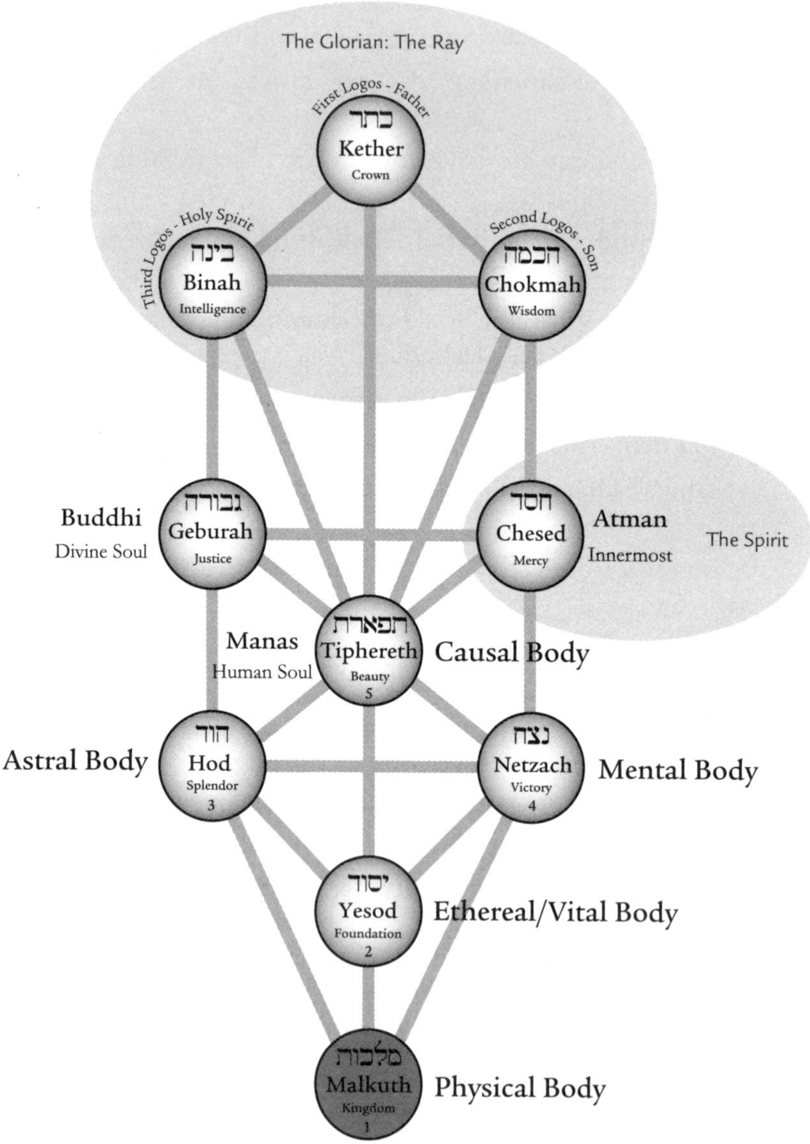

The Psyche and the Kabbalah

They saw the internal God of Krishnamurti and believed that he was Jesus of Nazareth; that was their mistake. What is most critical, is the damage that they perpetrated upon the Hindu boy. When a bodhisattva is told that his internal God is a Master, he becomes confused; he is damaged; he develops a complex.

The Hindu boy saw those instructors arguing among themselves because of him. Thus, the outcome was a psychological trauma for his human personality. Krishnamurti had a psychological trauma.

There is no doubt that the Theosophist clairvoyants did great damage to the Hindu boy. The Theosophist Hierarchs should have left the Hindu boy in peace. He would have developed himself freely in India. Then, his work would have been marvelous.

The great Buddha of Krishnamurti did not give his whole message, because his bodhisattva had a psychological trauma.

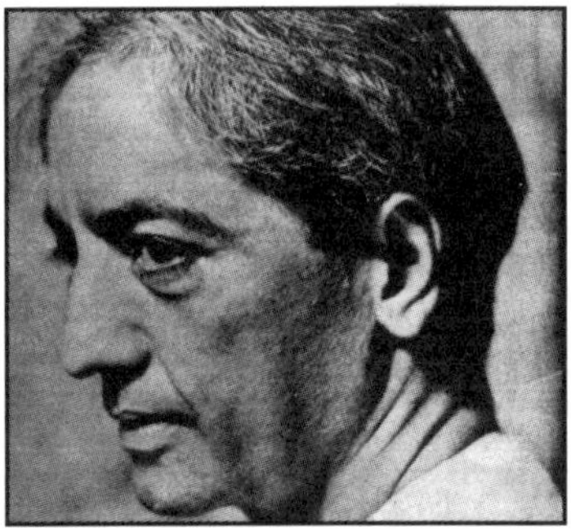

If we examine the doctrine of Krishnamurti, we see that the best of it is Buddhism. Unfortunately, he does not know the Christic Esotericism.

The Hindu body drank from the fountain of the Buddhist Gospel. It is a pity that he did not know the Christic Esotericism.

Later on, he mixed the Buddhist Philosophy with the Conventional Philosophy from the Western World.

Thus, the doctrine of Krishnamurti is the outcome of that mixture. The doctrine of Krishnamurti is Buddhism.

However, the doctrine of Aquarius is the outcome of the mixture of Buddhist Esotericism with Christic Esotericism.

The doctrine of Krishnamurti is Free Buddhism. However, the living fountain of that doctrine is the marvelous gospel of the Lord Buddha.

We are not against Krishnamurti; we only regret the fact that the Internal Buddha of that Hindu Philosopher could not give the whole message. That is all.

When a clairvoyant discovers that the Innermost (the Spirit) of someone is a Master, then it is best for that clairvoyant to be silent, in order not to damage that person.

When somebody knows that his inner being is a Master, he becomes filled with pride and arrogance. Fortunately, Krishnamurti learned how to be humble.

Fallen bodhisattvas also exist. These ones are worse than demons.

No one has to be told that his inner Being is a Master. The clairvoyant must be prudent. The clairvoyant must learn how to be silent.

The Spirit of someone could have achieved the degree of Master in some ancient reincarnation. The bodhisattva (Human Soul of the Master) could have fallen later on, thus now that Soul can live upon the path of evil.

The Master never falls. The one who falls is the bodhisattva (Human Soul) of the Master.

The clairvoyant must be prudent; thus, before announcing a new Master, he must wait with patience many years, in order to see how the person of flesh and bones, the terrestrial bodhisattva, behaves. The Master could be very great above; yet, the person of flesh and bones (bodhisattva) here below is dangerous.

In any case, *By their fruits you will know them.*

Madame Blavatsky stated that one of the greatest mysteries of occultism is the mystery of the double personality.

All the fights and errors of the Theosophical Society were the cause of the trauma of Krishnamurti. The Krishnamurti case is very important.

Dr. Steiner knew the Christic Mysteries. This is why he did not allow himself to be confused. Steiner was Gnostic.

Steiner did not accept that Krishnamurti was the reincarnation of Jesus Christ.

Many followed Steiner and many others Lady Besant.

The clairvoyant Steiner had a vast intellectual culture; this is why he did not fall into that mistake. Steiner was a true Rosicrucian Gnostic.

Chapter 24

The Mentally Obsessed One, the Client, the Succubus

Many cases of witchcraft are frequently presented before the tribunals.

Regarding witchcraft cases, the authorities laugh about them. They concretely judge common crimes. They completely exclude stories regarding warlocks, santeros, sorcerers, or whatever they want to call them.

The warlocks or black magicians, etc. already know that the authorities do not believe in their tenebrous science. When the Mentally Obsessed One, the Client, the Sorcerer, etc. have to answer in front of the authorities, they prefer to talk concretely about the exterior aspect of the crime, since they know by their own experience that the authorities do not believe in witchcraft, sorcery, etc., etc.

Internally, the warlocks consider the authorities as people who know very much. Yet, the warlocks know that regarding witchcraft or matters of sorcery, the authorities are absolutely ignorant.

This is the concept that the honest sorcerers have about the authorities, sorcerers who sincerely believe in their religion and in the power and efficacy of their rites.

False sorcerers also exist who only live from extortion; they exploit their neighbors' credulity. These false sorcerers are extortionists.

We are going to study the honest sorcerers.

We do not deny that the mentalist, the one who performs the obsession, the godfather, the incubus, etc. are ignorant people. It is logical that ignorance is the mother of all crimes. Yet, this problem cannot be resolved with corrective pedagogic treatments that are based on strictly conventional culture. Neither are these problems resolved with privation of liberty, nor with forced labor.

The sorcerer continues to be a sorcerer in jail or in exile, with conventional culture or without it. The sorcerer states, "These people know a lot, yet regarding my science, they do not know anything about it. My science is superior."

To that end, the instructive and corrective conventional systems, as well as the systems of penalization, are useless in order to reform sorcerers. Those ignorant people can only be reformed with a superior spiritual culture. Those cases can only be treated with corrective pedagogic treatments based on Theosophy, Rosicrucianism, Yogic Philosophy, etc., etc. Professors on these matters should be available with special reformatories in order to treat these cases.

Witchcraft is behind thirty percent of common crimes. However, the delinquents keep silence, because they know that the judges are skeptical and totally ignorant about matters of witchcraft.

Indeed, the judges have a conventional intellectual culture. Yet, they do not know anything about the science of sorcerers.

Only the study of Gnosis, Theosophy, Rosicrucianism, Yogic Philosophy, etc. can change the skepticism of the judges. This way, they will move more towards the populace's soul.

Forensic psychiatry can tremendously expand with these studies in order to explore profoundly the *causa causorum* of any crime.

The criminal responsibility before the tribunals has extremely deep roots, so deep that not even the psychoanalysis of Freud suspects it.

We must leave aside mental laziness and those prejudices that make us utter phrases like, "Oh but, what would people say if I study this?" or "What would people say, if I educate myself in this?" We must study Gnosis, Theosophy, Rosicrucianism, Yogic Philosophy, etc.

Occult wisdom is the fundamental depth of any science.

The great German doctor Arnold Krumm-Heller narrates in his *Rosicrucian Novel* the case of a warlock who was performing sorcery on a wretched woman. He was performing his sorcery through the medium of a used piece of cloth from his victim. The unhappy woman became deranged or better said, the warlock made her insane.

When Dr. Krumm-Heller denounced the former case to the authorities, they mocked him. Of course, this is why, based on this type of authoritative skepticism, the delinquents from sorcery can commit the most horrible crimes. The human law does not affect the warlocks, since they always shelter themselves under the skepticism of the judges.

Warlocks are pleased with the skepticism of the judges, since their skepticism is convenient for them. Yet, woe to them if the judges were to know about witchcraft.

A Russian scientist invented an electronic brain that is capable of registering the mental force of a human being. If someone gives a command to such an electronic device, then the apparatus collects his cerebral radiations. Then, such a device places in movement other different machines through its very complicated and difficult mechanism. This is how the reality of the force of thought has already been demonstrated.

Once, the scientists were laughing when listening to statements on mental force; yet now, in Russia, in order to move machines, instead of pressing automatic buttons, they are starting to utilize the mental force.

We do not deny that the Mentalist, the One who Obsesses, the Obsessed One, the Client, and the Succubus are of an oligophrenic type. They are ignorant fanatics who, while in their state of delirium, commit horrendous crimes. Yet, the reality is that such people are utilizing the mental force that is already demonstrated by that scientific Russian device.

Mental waves travel throughout space. Shortly, the scientists will invent antennas that will be capable of capturing mental waves using apparatuses similar to the radio that will translate mental waves into sound. At that time, no one will conceal his thoughts anymore.

Nevertheless, in this day and age, apparatuses capable of measuring mental waves already exist. Scientists measure mental waves based on micro-voltage.

Therefore, the hour in which the judges have to stop laughing and must start studying has arrived.

Victor Hugo said: "The one who laughs at what he does not know is an ignoramus who walks the path of idiocy."

Let us look at Hypnotism, for instance. Until a relatively short time ago, Hypnotism seemed to us to be related with sorcerers and skulls amidst foggy nights.

In this day and age, Hypnotism is already officially accepted by medical science in order to heal the sick. Clinics with scientific devices for Hypnotism exist. Sorcerers who utilize hypnotism in order to perform their criminal deeds also exist. This is already established in the penal code of many countries.

A sorcerer can give a person a mental suggestion during a hypnotic trance. The sorcerer can mentally suggest to a passive person and command him to execute a crime. Later on, that person, without knowing where or why, goes and executes the command given by the sorcerer. This is how horrendous and frightful crimes have been committed.

The sorcerers also use distinct "embos" that they place at the doors of their victims. When the authorities get their hands on one of those famous "embos," then the proverbial skeptical laugh of the judges is provoked. The people already know the skepticism of the judges. This is why the accused ones prefer to hide such famous "embos." The "embos" can be made with special powders, water, toasted corn, feathers, dolls, pieces of cloth with menstrual blood, etc., etc.

The force of thought lies in the depth of these famous "embos." The imagination of the sorcerer is exalted with the "embos." This is how he projects cerebral waves that are capable of damaging and killing his hated victims.

It so happens that many of those victims of witchcraft and "embos" fall into delirium of persecution; they feel threatened by the paranormal forces of the sorcerer. If the victim is hysteric and impulsive, he can then commit a hysterical homicide, an act of hysteria.

Many times, these types of criminals (who in their depth are victims) suffer "hysterical-epileptic" attacks.

Huxley, the materialistic scientist, accepted that many types of living beings populate the Ether (the Ultra).

The dialectic materialists reject the Ether; they state that only the electromagnetic energies exist; however, this is only a new name that is given onto the Ether.

Millions of microbes exist within a drop of water; this drop is infinite for them.

Beasts and monsters that the human being cannot perceive exist within the "Ultra-special." They cannot perceive them due to the distinct modifications of matter. Metaphysics and dialectical materialism know nothing about it.

The clairvoyant can perceive these types and forms of life (even if the materialists laugh about it). The ultra-micrometer can register up to the ten thousandth part of a millimeter.

An English doctor invented a lens with which the aura, the irradiation of the Astral Body, can be seen.

Soon, lenses with which the fourth dimension will be seen will exist. Then scholastic metaphysics and dialectic materialism will become ludicrous before the solemn verdict of the public consciousness.

At that time, we will see through those lenses the monsters and the larvae which obsess the minds of delinquents.

If the judges will laugh about it, then they will also have to laugh about microbes and renounce the microscope and vaccinations.

Logic invites us to think that if physical microbes that damage the physical body exist, mental microbes: larvae, incubae, succubae, basilisks, dragons, etc. that damage the mind must also exist.

These types of mental microbes will be visible for the whole world in a short time. Yesterday, the microscope was invented in order to see the physical microbes. Tomorrow, the Ultra-microscope will be invented in order to see the microbes from the Ultra-world.

If physical epidemics exist, moral epidemics, that is to say, immoral waves of suicide, thievery, violence, etc., etc., also exist. This can be confirmed in the cities.

Microbes are the agents of those epidemics, in both cases. Logic is logic.

The demon-possessed ones from Jatibonico, in which a whole family suffered the most strange and diverse mental disturbances, and the case of "Mama Coleta" mentioned in chapter sixteen of this book, are concrete cases of psychic obsession. These are cases of moral epidemics.

The active agents of those epidemics are from the Ultra, namely: trolls, larvae, incubae, evil spirits, etc., etc. These types of names awaken resistance in the skeptical materialist.

Let us not argue about terminology. If you like, baptize these lives from the Ultra with the name of Ultra-sensible microbes. I think this name will satisfy the skeptical materialist. Most of the time, we human beings argue over terminology. So let us agree with the former terms, and thereafter, let us continue analyzing the subject matter.

A trauma is what the skeptical materialists have in their psychological depth. The cause of that trauma is Roman Catholic dogmatism. They became disappointed by the Roman sect; thus, the outcome of their disappointment was a psychological trauma. They are the enemies of Hegel.

Now, anything that smells as spirituality, unconsciously seems, for these skeptical materialists, as being from the Roman Catholic Church. This is their psychological trauma.

So, you, skeptical materialists, let us inform you (in order for you to listen to us, aside from your traumatic and sick "I") that we are neither Catholics nor Materialists.

Yes, listen, we are neither Catholics nor Materialists; we are Gnostics. Gnosis signifies knowledge, wisdom.

Let us study then the Ultra-sensible microbes.

The sorcerer Barrueta mentally obsessed the unhappy clairvoyant medium woman from chapter sixteen. What? Does the term "sorcerer" bother you? Are you afraid to believe in sorcerers? Well then, be afraid also of microbes. What if we named the sorcerers microbes and the microbes sorcerers? It is just a matter of terminology, right? Then, why do we have to argue?

Let us analyze without pre-concepts. The medium and the whole family of the "Mama Coleta" case were obsessed by evil spirits, trolls, sorcerers, etc. (Ultra-sensible microbes that within a short time, when optics advance towards the Ultra, will become visible).

As a leper has his body invaded by the bacterium of Hansen, and a person with tuberculosis has his lungs invaded by the bacterium of Kock; likewise, the Ultra-sensible microbes can obsess the mind and direct a human being to commit a crime.

Two types of epidemics exist and two types of sicknesses exist, namely, the physical and the psychic.

Everything is reduced to the atom. The atom is a trio of matter, energy, and consciousness. We need to investigate how the atomic intelligences behave.

If no one accepted the microbes in the epoch of Pasteur, if they laughed at that sage because he was disinfecting the instruments of surgery, why is it so strange then that they laugh about us, the Gnostics, because we accept the existence of Ultra-sensible microbes?

These are just things of this epoch! Yet, when the science of optics advances, then they will be our best defenders. This is how the course of history has always been.

The famous "embos" from sorcerers are contaminated poisonous substances.

Those substances are true Ultra-microbe-carriers that can sensibly infect the organism of their victims and can lead them towards dementia and death. Even if the medical science of this century ignores this, later it will know it.

The sorcerers' "embos" are very dangerous, bacterium-carrier substances.

A psychic epidemic was the *causa causorum* of the "Mama Coleta" case.

Jails are filled with delinquents who are mentally sick. The Ultra-sensible microbes make the mind sick and conduce the human being to crime.

Millions of delinquents feel themselves to be innocent, and a mental prophylactic still does not exist for them, or offices for mental health, either. In this day and age, people speak abundantly about physical culture; yet, institutes for psychic culture are more necessary now than ever. We admit to the existence of air currents that are truly carriers of infectious bacteria. Yet, we ignore the existence of mental currents that are transmitters of Ultra-sensible microbes, capable of damaging, causing illness, and even killing their victims.

The "Mama Coleta" case is related with a mental infection that was transmitted by the mental currents of a sorcerer. His victims fell into jail and death; yet, he, the secret assassin, remained immune. He was not caught; he saved himself by hiding behind the skepticism of the judges.

The cases of psychic obsession must be studied by forensic psychiatry.

Jails are filled with mentally sick people. There is no doctor for those wretched ones. Thousand of delinquents are innocent.

Forensic psychiatry needs to be expanded.

A specific antidote exists for each sickness.

Sorcerers are not reformed with external culture. No sick person is cured with an incompatible remedy. We cannot cure typhus with remedies for measles. Each sickness needs its special antidote.

Sorcerers are reformed with their special antidote. That antidote for sorcerers is the occult wisdom, namely: Gnosis, Theosophy, Rosicrucianism, Yogic Philosophy, etc., etc.

It is obvious that when a delinquent is condemned, the evidence of the "corpus delicti" is required. To justify the "corpus delicti," in accordance with all the legal forms that are established by the codex of penal processes, is also necessary.

A human being cannot be condemned for the crime of black magic if the evidence of the "corpus delicti" is not known. Neither can he be condemned if the "corpus delicti" has not been justified in accordance with all the legal forms that are established by the codex of penal processes.

When a citizen is accused of the crime of black magic, when a citizen is accused as being a black magician, the "corpus delicti" must exist and that "corpus delicti," must have been rightly justified in accordance with the penal processes.

When a citizen is accused, when a citizen is designated a black magician without the "corpus delicti," without criminal antecedents, without judicial evidences, then the accuser falls into the crime of calumny and defamation of character.

People who dedicate themselves to the studies of Occultism, Theosophy, Rosicrucianism, Gnosis, Yogic Philosophy, etc., etc., constantly fall into the crimes of calumny, public slander, defamation of character, etc., etc.

Those people must take care of their tongue, because frequently they fall into the crimes of calumny, public slander, defamation of character, etc., etc.

To asseverate that such a fellow or such a lady is a black magician is a crime of calumny, public slander, and defamation of character. The spiritual brethren should learn how to control their tongues.

For by their fruits you will know them. Each person is known through his deeds. A citizen cannot be a black magician without criminal antecedents.

A lady and a gentleman who accomplish their duties as mother or father and pay their debts, have never killed, stolen, slandered, etc. cannot be black magicians.

The skeptics of materialism laugh about all of these things. Therefore, leaving aside the fanaticism of the materialistic sect, we, the Gnostics, say the following: "The one who laughs at what he does not know is an ignoramus who walks the path of idiocy."

Therefore, when a scientist mocks Asian Yoga and Esoteric Buddhism, he becomes an ignoramus who walks the path of idiocy.

Thanks to the practical science of the occident, technical advancement has been achieved as well as a revolution in forensic psychiatry.

The practical, experimental, and demonstrative science of the occident allows us to place physical matter at our service.

The practical, experimental, and demonstrative science of oriental Yoga allows us to awaken the senses of internal perception. We can see, hear, touch, and feel the fourth dimension.

When a human being expands his senses of perception, he then receives new scientific information that increases his wisdom. The esoteric science is the fundamental basis of nature.

When the occidental and oriental science are completely joined, then the human being will reach a new integral and total culture, free of fanatical sectarisms.

In this day and age, the science of criminology is found stagnant because of the superstitions of the fanatic materialistic sect.

Chapter 25

The Alienated Ones

It is impossible to know the fundamental cause of any mental disequilibrium without expanding Psychiatry with Theosophy, Rosicrucianism, Hermeticism, Yogic Philosophy, and high Gnostic Esotericism.

This is how the expanded psychiatry can discover and cure the alienated ones.

We knew the case of a young woman who fell into a state of furious madness. This young lady was interned for six months in a mental health center. There, she was submitted to the classic medical treatments with the famous electric shocks, diet, etc. Nonetheless, everything was a complete and absolute failure.

That lady, when in shock, was writhing like a serpent; she was foaming through her mouth while pronouncing incoherent words, etc., etc.

We, the students of expanded psychiatry, purposed ourselves to profoundly study this case. Thus, we found the following symptoms:

Indeed, she had abnormal ideas related with strange psychopathic deliriums. She had deliriums of persecution. She believed herself to be wanted by the police and condemned to death. She felt herself accused and wanted for robbery, etc.

When exploring the psyche of this sick woman, we found anguish during her delirium and a choleric physiognomy. Sometimes she was filled with terror and, at other times, melancholy.

It appears among the antecedents of her social evolution that during her infancy, adolescence, and youth she developed normally in her home and in school without anything strange having occurred to her.

She did not present symptoms of bruises, wounds, or anything of the sort.

Her psychopathic personality was of a totally schizoid type and she was introverted in an abnormal way.

The great sages are introverted; yet, they are not schizoids. They are normally introverted individuals.

The schizoid attitude of this sick lady belongs to the hyper-sensible and hyper-emotive type.

The type of schizoid personality described by Nretschmer is a difficult exploration for psychoanalysis. The interior life of those subjects is a constant mystery.

The schizoid type is hermetic, contradictory, sometimes very sensible, charitable and tender, yet other times, very cold, cruel and indifferent.

This sick lady had a certain self-aggressiveness with a suicide complex.

The schizoid constitution, the depressive tendency, the suicide complex with deliriums of persecution, and anguish presented a very complicated diagnostic.

Thus, before this case, medical science capitulated, and the sages with all of their science failed.

Nevertheless, we, the students of the expanded psychiatry, did not surrender. We proposed to study her case. We investigated her hereditary antecedents, and we did not find any insane or schizoid person among her ancestors.

The study of her brain and the general clinical analysis did not present any strange anomaly.

This problem was very difficult. Everything was enigmatic. The family of the sick woman had to take her out of the mental health center. Medical science had failed with this case.

What is most intriguing about this sick woman is that during her deliriums, in which she felt to be condemned to death, she was trying to free herself from some imaginary ropes. She believed herself to be tied up with ropes. She was holding the imaginary ropes and struggling to liberate herself from them in order to escape death. Materialistic science could not cure that case. The sick woman became an enigma for the doctors.

The scientific investigations of the erudite: the materialistic studies, the rigorous corroborations of the different chemical, physical, biochemical, physiological, etc., phenomena are not complete, because the erudite have not studied Gnosis. They do not know about *Kundalini Yoga* by Sivananda. They do not know about *Jnana Yoga* by Vivekananda. They have not studied *The Subtle Laws of Nature* by the famous Hindustani sage Rama Prasad. They have not exercised themselves with the Tattvic powers. They do not know about the esoteric and endoteric anthropogenesis and cosmogenesis. They do not know anything about Occult Anatomy nor about the Law of Karma, etc., etc. To that end, the materialistic science is incomplete and is a failure. It is only a building without a foundation. It is enough to push that building a little in order to convert it into minute sediment!

The most critical aspect of this matter is not the materialistic science but the fanaticism of the partisans of the Dialectic Materialism.

The fanatic partisans of the Dialectic Materialism do not accept anything that disagrees with their materialistic pontificates and priests (the tricksters of science). Those sectarian fanatics do not want to recognize other methods for investigation and scientific corroboration. They want to recognize only their authoritative pontificates and priests. They believe themselves to have the last word of knowledge; they are convinced that no one knows more than they do.

To that end, the geographic east and the cultural east, namely: Tibet, Grand Tartary, China, Siam, Mongolia, etc. do not exist for the fanatic partisans of Dialectic Materialism, because they believe that they are the center of the universe and no one knows more than they do. They think that everything that does not belong to them is worthless, and only what belongs to them is of value, because they think themselves to be wise, powerful, omnipotent, etc.

What is most ludicrous about these sectarians of the Dialectic Materialism is that they do not want to see beyond their noses. They put a limit to life based on their little intelligence. They seem to be like the medieval people who believed that beyond the Cape of Finisterre there was no more land and this was the limit of the earth. However, when Christopher Columbus talked about his projected adventure, they qualified him as a madman. Thus, if the Queen of Spain, Isabel la Catolica, had never helped Columbus in his intrepid enterprise, then the Spaniards would never have discovered America. Another intrepid one would have come ahead of them.

The sectarian materialists, who do not see beyond dogmatic procedures, look like the caterpillar that believes that the leaf where it lives is the whole. The caterpillar ignores that above and below that leaf there exists many other leaves from the tree where it lives. Likewise, the sectarian materialist ignores that other worlds exist above and below his external sensorial perceptions. What is worse is that those sectarian materialists not only ignore, but moreover, they ignore that they ignore. They are twofold ignorant.

We, the Gnostics, do not reach the point of affirming that scientific materialistic investigation is useless. What we, the Gnostics, condemn is the fanaticism of the materialistic sect.

It is logical that the scientific investigation of the phenomena of matter is useful to the human being. Nevertheless, the materialistic science is not the whole science. Neither are the rigorous procedures of investigation and scientific corroboration from the occidental world and from the materialistic sages the only ones.

Everything must be in its own place. We cannot study astronomy with a microscope, nor can we study microbes with a telescope.

The Gnostic Rosicrucian sage knows the systems of investigation from the East and the West.

The worlds of Ultra and of the Astral Body of the human being exist; they are a tremendous reality.

The physical material world exists and it is also a tremendous reality.

We investigate the worlds of the Ultra and of the Astral Body with the systems and methods of the Yogis of Hindustan.

We study the physical world with the methods of occidental investigation.

Both systems complement and harmonize each other. Both systems will give us in the future a new culture and a new civilization, highly mystical and formidably technical and scientific.

The human being of the future will place matter under his service. The machines will serve the community. The human being will not be a victim of any machine.

Medical science, astronomy, technology, aviation, industry, etc., etc., will liberate the spirit from slavery, from material labor.

The human being of the future will be endowed with illuminated intellect. The human being of the future will be endowed with the powers of clairvoyance, and, nonetheless, he will have gigantic scientific and technical advancements. He will be highly spiritual and marvelously intellectual.

So, the fanatical secularism of the partisans of the Dialectic Materialism is conservative, retarded, and anti-revolutionary.

The alienated ones increase in number every day, and doctors cannot cure them, because they do not know the Mental Body. If the materialistic sages would study the Oriental Yogic philosophy, then they would know the Mental Body. That way, they could cure thousands of madmen who live without hope.

A clairvoyant student of expanded psychiatry proposed to investigate the past reincarnation of the young alienated lady who was discarded by the materialists.

The outcome of the clairvoyant investigation gave as the clue. The "values" that were reincarnated in that young lady were incarnated in her past life as a thief, a road cracksman.

That thief, road cracksman, bandit, was searched for by the police and executed during the epoch of Don Porfirio Diaz (Mexico). The bandit was tied to a tree, and thereafter he was shot.

Now, we had a clue about her sickness. Then, we could explain to ourselves about the imaginary ropes and the delirium of persecution. The anguish concerning death of the mad young lady was no longer an enigma for us. The whole problem was resolved.

Death's impressions had remained engraved in the subconsciousness of her reincarnating ego. These were the same values of the executed bandit. The memories were deposited within the subconsciousness of the young lady. These values revived in her consciousness the whole terrible anguish of that horrible tragic drama. The outcome was her madness that the materialistic sages could not cure.

The commotion was so terrible for this young lady that her Mental Body was fissured. Many malignant atoms penetrated through those gaps of her Mental Body and infected her brain, forcing this sick young lady to perform absurd things.

Even though the materialistic sages are bothered by our procedures, we cannot deny that we were obligated to utilize Taumaturgy in order to heal the sick lady.

After six months of treatment with occult medicine, the sick young lady returned to her senses, she became radically cured.

This was a great victory for Taumaturgy and expanded psychiatry.

Mental health centers are filled with furious or passive maniacs.

The sickness of the alienated ones is in the Mental Body.

The Mental Body has its sicknesses and its symptoms.

It is necessary to study the Mental Body and its sicknesses.

The Third Logos closed the wounds of the Mental Body; this is how the sick lady was healed absolutely.

Jails are filled with alienated criminals.

Many normal delinquents have had a passing disturbing moment, thus they commit crimes in those instants of terrible over-excitement.

Sometimes, malaria fever produces furious deliriums whose final outcome is crime. The so-called hallucinations that are produced during fever states are legitimate perceptions of the Ultra.

Commonly, delirium is observed during scarlet fever, small pox, malaria fever, typhus, etc.

Any alteration, any transitory mental disturbance, any perturbation of the psychic functions, even the ones that are the outcome of infected deliriums, can conduce to crime.

The subjective sensorial impressions, which occur during somnolence or lethargy in the course of pathologic processes, are not illusion. Those impressions are legitimate ultra-sensible perceptions that enclose the clues of sickness.

Expanded psychiatry studies these perceptions in order to find the clue that will allow us to cure a sick person. In the course of a situational reaction with a transitory mental disturbance, a person can commit homicide, robbery, etc., etc.

Anthropometry cannot give us an explanation of intimate causes of a situational reaction with transitory mental disturbance and crime. The somatoscopic and the somasometric characteristics cannot give with logical exactitude the most intimate clues of a situational reaction with a transitory mental disturbance and crime.

Many times, the somatoscopic and the somasometric characteristics of assassins and thieves are found in normal citizens who do not register judicial antecedents.

Only by profoundly exploring the depths of the mind can we discover the secret origins of a situational reaction, a transitory mental disturbance, and its related crime.

Secret factors from the infraconsciousness, subconsciousness, or unconsciousness can be the cause of those mental transitory disturbances and of those types of situational reactions that carry any man or any woman towards crime.

The ultra-sensible microbes invade the mind and produce those situational reactions, transitory mental disturbances, and common crimes.

Our affirmations might appear absurd to the materialists. Yet, when did our affirmations not appear absurd to them? Were they perhaps the same ones who mocked about Pasteur and microbes? Is it then so strange now that they mock about our ultra-sensible and hyper-sensible microbes?

Those microbes are already classified, namely: Incubi, Succubi, Basilisks, Dragons, Elementals, Larvae, Tantric Entities, etc., etc.

If you materialists want to see and analyze them, then get a special lens. This special lens is clairvoyance. Do the perceptions of clairvoyance bother you? Well then, it is very clear that you are fanaticized! A psychological trauma is what lies in the depths of the materialists' fanaticism. So, in regards to this type of trauma, within these types of minds, everything that relates to spirituality provokes a psychological resistance. Therefore, the materialists' minds have a psychopathic sickness indeed.

We will radically change the present situation of the world with an in-depth integral culture on a spiritual, social, and scientific basis.

AGLA and the powerful Gnostic Movement, as well as Sivananda Aryabarta Ashrama, are the powerful integral cultural lever with which we can revolutionize the world and give it a total change.

The Gnostic Movements grant us the Esoteric Christic Wisdom. The Gnostic Wisdom will grant us a powerful intellectual, social, and revolutionary culture.

Sivananda Aryabarta Ashrama teaches us a rigorously analytical and tremendously scientific Yoga.

Our esoteric wisdom endures the most rigorous inductive and deductive analysis. In this day and age, the problem of the alienated ones is very critical. We can resolve this problem only with expanded psychiatry.

First of all, we need to free the mind from the conservative ideas of materialism and to enter deeply into the studies of AGLA.

Chapter 26

Total Revolution and Partial Revolution

The order of the factors does not alter the product.

The partial revolution is not total revolution.

The order of economical and political factors can be modified without the vital product suffering any change. Life continues with all of its pains. Partial revolution changes the order of the factors, yet it does not alter the vital product. Human beings continue mutually tormenting each other.

We Gnostics do not like partial revolution; we want total revolution. We can have total revolution only by dissolving the "I," the myself, the ego.

The "I" sabotages and damages the revolutionary order.

The "I" forms conflicts amidst the revolutionary orders.

The "I" wants to escalate, to rise, to show off, and to make itself noticed everywhere.

The "I" exploits; the "I" steals; the "I" cheats; the "I" slanders; the "I" calumniates and makes turbid the waters of revolution.

The "I" conflicts and forms problems in public education, in agrarian matters, in commercial transactions, in the public ministry, etc.

The truth comes to us when we dissolve the "I." When we dissolve the "I," we think with a consciousness of multitudes. We do not affirm the "I" when we dissolve the "I," instead, we affirm the pronoun "We."

When we attain the total revolution, each one of us becomes a perfect government.

Who wants to govern when each one of us is already a perfect government?

This is total, integral, absolute revolution.

When the "I" will be dissolved, all governments will disappear, because they will be useless.

The "I" is the origin of crime and pain.

The "I" created pain.

The Universal Spirit of Life did not create pain.

The "I" is the author of pain.

The "I" is Satan. Satan created pain.

If what is divine did not create pain, if Satan created pain, then pain is useless, absurd, and stupid.

Those who affirm that through pain we reach perfection are deifying Satan (the "I").

Whosoever loves pain is masochistic and satanic.

We decapitate the "I" only with the Arcanum A.Z.F.

We dissolve the "I" only with a profound creative comprehension.

Every human being has formed some opinion about the Truth. Every religion of every school has its own opinion about the Truth.

Human beings search for the Truth; they adore the Truth.

We, the Gnostics, state: *Know the Truth and the Truth shall make you free.* This is how total revolution will exist.

However, we warn you that no one can search for what he does not know.

The Truth is the unknowable from moment to moment.

The Truth comes to us without us searching for it.

The Truth comes to us when the "I" is dead.

Pain cannot conduce us towards the Truth, because pain belongs to Satan.

Only the Arcanum A.Z.F. and profound creative comprehension can lead us towards the Truth.

Every desire originates ideas. Every idea transforms itself into projects. Every project is desire. Projects conduce us towards crime.

Projects are true monsters that devour the neighbor, and in the end, they swallow their progenitor. This is how we become victims of our own inventions.

Desire is the origin of crime.

Desire is the origin of pain.

The delinquent enjoys when his desire is satisfied.

The delinquent suffers when his desire is frustrated.

Every human being is a delinquent even if he is not in jail.

If we comprehend the process of desire, we then dissolve the "I." When the "I" is dissolved, the origin of crime is finished. Total revolution exists when the "I" is dissolved.

You must transmute desire into willpower. This is how you will finish with desire.

When the sexual desire is transmuted into willpower, it becomes the flaming fire that victoriously ascends throughout the spinal medulla.

Every desire can be transmuted into light and fire.

Transmute desire into light; thus, the "I" will dissolve as a fatuous diabolic flame. This is how total revolution will exist.

Desire becomes extinguished when we transmute it.

We can transmute every desire based on creative comprehension only.

Desire is the fundamental matter of every crime.

The three most dangerous crimes are anger, greed, and lust. Anger is the violent outcome of frustrated desire. Greed is desire of accumulating. Lust is sexual desire.

Anger can be transmuted into sweetness. Greed can be transmuted into charity. Lust can be transmuted into love.

When the human being does not respect the life of his neighbor, he overestimates very much his own desire; this is how he kills.

When the human being steals, it is because he has the desire of accumulation, or he desires what he does not have.

The impurity of the mind is the dog of desire.

To lie is the desire of falsifying the truth.

Gossip and slander are frustrated desire or overestimation of one's own desire.

When someone feels himself frustrated in his own desires, he then gossips against his neighbor.

When someone overestimates his own Psychological "I," he then gossips against his neighbor.

The one who takes a false oath and the one who blasphemes against the divine overestimates his own desires too much.

Idle conversations are children of desire.

The one who envies, covets what he does not have. The one who covets is envious of his neighbor.

When someone covets, he desires. When someone envies, he covets what he does not have and feels distress because of his neighbor's goods.

Malice is accumulated desire. Hatred and resentment are frustrated desire.

Ignorance is the mother of desire. Desire of killing is transmuted into the science for healing and giving life. Desire of stealing is transmuted into altruism and charity.

Mental impurity is transmuted into chastity.

Desire of lying is transmuted into words of truth.

Desire of gossip and slander are transmuted into words of wisdom and love.

Desire of blasphemy and prejudice are transmuted into supreme veneration and adoration to the divine.

Desire and pleasure of idle conversations are transmuted into sublime silence and words of wisdom.

The frustrated desire of envy is transmuted into intimate happiness for our neighbor's goods.

The accumulative desire of greed is transmuted into the happiness of giving everything, even one's life, for the love of this suffering humanity.

The rottenness of malice is transmuted into the innocence of the child.

Anger, rancor, and hatred are distinct forms of desire that are transmuted into supreme sweetness, infinite pardon, and supreme love.

We must transmute all thoughts, words, and actions of desire into wisdom and love.

This is how we annihilate the "I."

That which is Non-temporal, the Eternal One, the Truth, the Inner Christ, comes to us when we annihilate the "I."

The only way to dissolve the "I" is by annihilating desire.

The only way to annihilate desire is by transmuting it. When a superior law transcends an inferior law, the superior law washes away the inferior law.

The science of transmutations is called Alchemy.

The basic foundation of Alchemy is the Arcanum A.Z.F.

Mind, heart, and sex are the perfect triangle of Holy Alchemy.

The struggle is terrible: brain against sex, sex against brain, and even more terrible and painful, heart against heart. You know this!

Many are those who blaspheme against the divine life, against God. They accuse the unknowable and divine of being the cause of all their sufferings and pains.

The great divine life has nothing to do with all the errors of the "I."

Any man or woman desires something; thereafter, they form their plans and projects. These plans and projects are very beautiful when they think about them; yet, the problems come when they want to fulfill them. When our plans are fulfilled we say, "God is very good to me, as he granted me what I desired." Yet, when those plans and projects fail, then the desire is frustrated and the devotee feels himself disappointed. He then blames God and blasphemes against the Eternal One. However, if they are Occultists or Theosophists, etc., etc., then they blame the Lords of Karma, or they blaspheme against them.

This is how humanity is!

People do not want to realize that what is Divine is absolute happiness and it has nothing to do with pain.

The "I" creates its own pain. The "I" is Satan.

Those who convert pain into a mysticism are masochists.

Pain ends when we dissolve the "I."

Total revolution exists when we dissolve the "I."

We annihilate the "I" based on alchemical operations only.

The incessant transmutations of Alchemy are performed in exact arithmetical operations.

Many masochistic students of Occultism, Theosophy, etc., etc., consider misery, pain and even sickness as an inexhaustible fountain of light and wisdom. Those wretched people adore the "I." Those people are Satanic.

God or that which is God, the Divinity, is happiness, peace, and abundance.

Misery and pain belong to Satan.

Other people await believing that through evolution and time they will one day attain perfection. Those people are even worse, because they want to perpetuate Satan throughout the centuries. They are worse, because they want to perfect Satan (Satan is the "I").

Satan enjoys when he reincarnates in order to satisfy his desires.

Satan enjoys when he gets more experience. The experiences of life complicate and strengthen the "I."

While his adolescence, youth, and maturity pass away, the innocent and beautiful child gains experiences that complicate him and finally transform him into a sly, malicious, distrustful, etc., old man.

The innocent human being of eighteen millions of years ago is now the human being of cabarets and of the atomic bomb, the human being of peculation and crime.

This is what the evolution of the "I" is. It is a complication and a fortification of the myself. It is the projection of error throughout the centuries.

Therefore, evolution ends when the "I" is dissolved. This is what total revolution is.

The Absolute does not know itself. The Absolute needs to know itself.

Each super-divine atom needs to know itself in order to have consciousness of its own happiness. Unconscious happiness is not happiness.

The human being, in his last synthesis, is just a super-divine atom from the Abstract Absolute Space. That atom is known by the Kabbalists with the name of **Ain Soph**.

It is urgent to know that the Ain Soph sends its Spirit to the world of matter with the purpose of acquiring that which is called Self-cognizance of its own happiness.

When the Spirit, after having passed through the mineral, plant, and animal states of consciousness, attains the human state, it can return into the Ain Soph to fuse with It.

This is how the Ain Soph becomes conscious of its own happiness.

Unfortunately, the human being allows himself to be confused by matter and by the fatal voices of desire. This is how the "I" is born.

The worst disgrace is the continuity of the "I." Satan complicates himself through reincarnation.

Satan suffers the consequences of his own errors through reincarnation (Karma).

Satan is born in time and dies in time. Satan is time.

To want to perfect Satan is an absurdity.

To want to become liberated with time is the same as to adore Satan.

That which is God, the Divine, the Truth, is non-temporal.

The human being organizes mystical schools with the great pain of Satan.

The human being converts pain into a mysticism. This is masochism.

We created the complicated theory of evolution based on a mistake.

The human being committed a mistake when he ate the forbidden fruit. This is how the "I" was born.

The forbidden fruit that Adam ate was sex.

Since then, the error continues reincarnating.

This is how pain continues.

We dissolve the "I" only through incessant transmutations. This is how evolution ends.

This is total revolution.

The economical and political revolution is partial revolution.

We need total revolution.

After the absolute death of the "I," the Spirit of the human being returns unto his interior star that has always smiled upon him. That star is a super-divine atom from the Abstract Absolute Space.

The spirit of the human being is the ray of that interior star.

The horrible dragon of desire trapped that ray.

Therefore, when the ray liberates itself from the horrible beast of desire, he then returns into his interior star. This is how the star becomes conscious of its own happiness.

The ray returns into its star by climbing the symbolic ladder of Jacob. In its return, the ray acquires angelic, archangelic, seraphic, etc., etc., types of consciousness.

Therefore, the divine hierarchies are the outcome of tremendous interior revolutions.

Partial revolution is another type of pain.

We need total revolution.

Total revolution is supreme happiness.

Chapter 27

Intellectual Criminology

Intellectual criminology is so profound and complex that we would need millions of volumes in order to study this single subject; therefore, we will touch on a few points only.

Intellectual criminology is found in books, magazines, bull fighting arenas, movie theaters, pamphlets, etc., etc.

Pornographic magazines that prostitute the minds of male and female youngsters exist in different countries.

When a pornographic representation reaches the mind, the unconsciousness traps that representation and elaborates its conceptual content.

The conceptual content elaborated by the unconsciousness is the exact outcome of the quality of the representation.

The psychological "I" traps that representation within the depths of the unconsciousness of the mind and elaborates its conceptual content with it.

The conceptual content is translated as semi-conscious images within the world of the cosmic mind. These are the effigies of the Mental World.

The psychological "I" fornicates and commits adultery with those images within the plane of the cosmic mind.

This is what the prostitution of the mind is.

Nocturnal pollutions (wet dreams) are the morbid outcome of the prostitution of the mind.

Magazines for the failures also exist.

In the magazines for the failures, women announce themselves. They solicit for a husband who is short, fat, skinny, with money, etc., etc. Many young ladies are following that ultramodern example. This is what mental prostitution is.

The outcome of this mental prostitution is critical. The interchange of letters begins. They start falling in love with someone whom they do not know and they start projecting plans.

Yet, in the end, on the day when the couples encounter, failure is the inevitable outcome.

Ladies who have never been prostitutes, honorable and distinguished young ladies, allow themselves to be cheated by modernism and fall into the crime of mental prostitution.

If a clairvoyant were to study in the Mental Plane the announcements of love of all of those magazines, he then will see houses of prostitution. Each announcement of love corresponds within the Mental World to a horrible mental bedroom of a whorehouse.

Every clairvoyant is astonished when seeing those whorehouses from the Mental Plane.

A prostitute, lying down, is found within each bedroom of those horrible dens.

Men enter and leave from those bedrooms.

Each announcement of the magazine corresponds to one of those bedrooms.

The woman who placed the announcement is lying down in her bedroom.

This is what the prostitution of the Mental Plane is.

True love has nothing to do with those whorehouses of the Mental Plane.

Thousands of young and distinguished ladies are perverting themselves with those types of magazines.

True love begins always with a flash of delectable sympathy. It is substantiated with the force of tenderness and it is synthesized in infinite supreme adoration.

True love is natural, without artifices, as the love of birds, as the love of the fish of the immense sea, as the love of the savage creature from the impenetrable jungle.

Another intellectual crime is "bull fighting."

The first critical symptoms are shown among those women who in their emotional climax hurl even their intimate underwear or pantyhose to the Torero.

It is ludicrous to see women's shoes or any type of dressing garments falling down into the arena.

Those women look insane.

Violent emotion causes transitory mental disturbances. The violent emotion is a function of the instinctive "I."

Antisocial and highly criminal acts are the outcome of violent emotions. Violent emotions originate instantaneous psychic traumas.

The violent sensation transmitted by the Torero, the bullfighter, produce internal criminal reflexes within the depths of the mind.

The mental criminal reflexes evolve within the psychobiological field of the human infraconsciousness.

Internal criminal reflexes that evolve within the field of the infraconsciousness are the secret causes of criminal sadism.

Three types of emotions exist: Light, Optima, and Puissant.

The first one does not achieve the total alteration of the mind.

The second one places the sensual imagination into activity, inhibiting intellectual analysis. This is when we see the hysteric-emotive episodes, as those from the black masses of the Middle Ages. The hysteric-emotive episodes from bull fighting arenas and those from black masses during the Middle Ages are similar.

We find shouts without control in both cases; women hurl their dressing garments, intellectual analysis disappears, etc.

The third type, puissant emotion, annuls any type of reasoning and the victim falls into the state of coma or stupor.

Many times, within the bull fighting arenas, some very sensible people fall unconscious, senseless. During the black masses, many women with an evolving epileptic type of emotion, extremely hyper-emotive, fall on the floor senseless with epileptic convulsions. Then, everybody is satisfied, because they consider these women to be possessed by the devil.

We believe that people who are mediums are easily obsessed by hyper-sensible microbes: astral larvae, incubi, elementals, and every type of inferior entity of the Astral Plane.

Mental disturbances of traumatic origin are the fatal outcome of violent emotions.

Bull fighting arenas have their origin in Pagan Rome.

Later, those barbarian circuses planted their roots in Spain.

It is lamentable that such a sad spectacle had been transplanted to Latin America.

Animal protection societies should fight against those types of bloody spectacles.

The fault of this type of spectacle falls upon the Roman Catholic Church one hundred percent. That Roman Sect is the intellectual author of that criminal spectacle, because that sect is the one that denied onto the animals the legitimate right of having an immortal soul.

The Torero believes that the animal has no soul. This is why they stab the picks within the afflicted flesh of the innocent victim without ever feeling charity or mercy.

The Torero is an executioner of innocents.

The Torero is worse than the sanguinary tiger of Bengal, because the Torero does not kill by a savage instinct of self-defense nor to satiate his hunger.

The Torero kills innocent animals in order to entertain the multitudes, who are avid and thirsty for blood and pleasure. The Torero is similar to the Roman Gladiator who after impaling the heart of his victim exclaimed, "Hail, Caesar!"

The word "animal" comes from the word *anima* (Soul). The word *anima* remains just by taking the letter "L" from the word "animal."

The animal is an *anima*. The *anima* of the animal is an innocent and beautiful elemental.

Every atom is a trio of matter, energy and consciousness.

The consciousness of every atom is always an intelligent elemental.

If the materialists are not capable of seeing those elementals, it is because they still do not know the scientific procedures that allow us to see them.

We have special methods in order to see those creatures.

Indeed, the atom is a truly infinitely small planetary system.

Those planetary systems of the atoms are formed by ultra-atomic ternaries that spin around their centers of gravitation.

The atom with its Alpha, Beta, and Gamma rays is a trio of matter, energy and consciousness.

The monistic doctrine of the Haeckelian materialist states that force and matter are the same thing. The materialist Haeckel asseverates that consciousness is latent in everything that exists and "he states" that we must search for it within our brain cells.

We, the Gnostics, go further beyond, because we know Occult Anatomy and the Astral Body.

The Cosmic Consciousness reflects itself in the whole panorama of the universe.

We know that Cosmic Consciousness exerts upon force and that the latter acts upon matter.

The coordinates of every biologic, physiologic, atomic, etc., etc. phenomena are intelligent. Every directive intelligence is conscious.

We cannot admit bio-mechanic phenomena without conscious coordinates.

You can be sure that the fanatic, conservative, and retarded materialist dogmatically rejects the former affirmations.

The psychological trauma of the fanatics of Dialectic Materialism is reactionary.

The organism of the animal is a synthesis of matter, energy, and consciousness.

The animal consciousness is an intelligent elemental.

The mineral, plant, animal, and human being have soul.

That soul is the Cosmic Consciousness. Only one soul exists; this is the Cosmic Consciousness. That is the *Anima Mundi* of Plato. The Great Consciousness is co-essential with Abstract Absolute Space.

You can call that great consciousness God, Allah, Parabrahman or whatever you like; in the end it does not matter a bit.

What is important is to comprehend the reality of the Great Consciousness.

Human words are smoke that cloud the starry heaven of the spirit.

What is important is the Great Reality.

The Torero who assassinates the unhappy beast commits a horrible crime against the great Universal Fraternity.

We, all beings, are one within the Universal Spirit of Life.

The hunter who kills his minor brothers (the animals) commits also the cowardly crime of fratricide.

The boxer who punches his brother in order to entertain the multitudes is also a fratricide.

The wrestling fighters, boxers, the toreros, the sly and perverse hunters, etc., etc., are assassins.

The intellectual author of all of those crimes is the Catholic Religion.

Chapter 28

Bellicose Psychosis

The press, radio, magazines, etc., have created the state of bellicose psychosis.

The Gnostic Movement, AGLA and Sivananda Aryavarta Ashrama fight against the bellicose necroneurosis.

Bellicose psychosis evolving within the human infra-consciousness finally converts itself into violence, hatred, and war. Bellicose psychosis originates sicknesses.

A soldier became blind while in the middle of a battle in the Second World War. The cause of his blindness was his self-culpability. The man saw a hand grenade coming; thus, he cast himself down to the ground and sheltered behind a boulder.

If he had warned his comrades, they would have not died; therefore, he felt guilty and became blind.

When the doctors examined him, they did not find any wound in his eyes.

The psychiatrist who hypnotized him could cure him because he discovered the cause. The psychiatrist commanded the man to see and he saw.

Naturally, the psychiatrist had to persuade him with good arguments in order for the man to forget his culpability.

Gnosis is promoting the advent of a new civilization and culture.

Gnosis unites all philosophical and spiritual schools, all religions, and sects, in order to study on a round table all the economical and social problems of humanity. Gnosis works, longing for the day in which each citizen becomes truly free and just.

Gnosis is a universal revolutionary movement that fights for the advent of the new Aquarian Era.

Cultural-spiritual labor must replace bellicose propaganda.

Gnosis performs in many parts of the world a gigantic cultural-spiritual labor.

Bellicose propaganda is destructive and dangerous.

The human being must resolve all of his problems without wars and without bellicose propaganda.

Chapter 29

Paranoia

The paranoid appears normal.

The reasoning and completely lucid madness is named paranoia.

Great personages are always in danger of being assassinated by paranoids.

Many presidents and statesmen have been assassinated by paranoids.

Commonly, the paranoid is a delirious one with false ideas.

We knew the case of a paranoid Rosicrucian boss. That man intended to monopolize the Rosicrucian Science. He was a paranoid with deliriums of grandeur. He considered himself as the unique priest of the truth.

The distrust and pride of that Rosicrucian paranoid were tremendous.

The truth is the unknowable from moment to moment.

However, that Rosicrucian paranoid was convinced of being the absolute owner of the truth.

He believed that he knew the truth.

Many are the Occultist, Theosophist Rosicrucians who become paranoids. Every Mystic-paranoid considers himself as the very incarnation of the truth.

The "I" cannot recognize the truth, because the "I" has not experienced the truth.

We can only recognize what we know; yet, we cannot recognize what we do not know.

The "I" does not know the truth. The "I" is born in time and dies in time.

The "I" is time itself.

The truth does not belong to the "I," because the truth is not of time.

The truth is non-temporal; it is eternal.

The paranoid has deliriums about the truth and believes that he has the truth.

The human being can rack his brain searching for the truth, yet he will not find it.

The paranoid believes that he has the truth. Indeed, he only projects opinions about the truth. The mind is bottled up within the "I."

Some stubborn people say that God exists; others say that God or the truth does not exist.

Those who say that the truth exists and those who deny it are both stubborn.

To affirm or to deny the existence of the truth is opinion.

Every opinion is a mental projection of the "I," of the myself.

Every affirmation and negation of the truth does not increase or take away an atom from the infinite.

Those who search for the truth are imbeciles, because no one can search what he does not know.

The Occultist, Theosophist, etc., paranoid believes that he can find and recognize the truth.

A person can never recognize another person whom he has never known.

Therefore, no one can recognize the truth, because no one has ever known it.

Let us not talk about the truth. It is better to talk about Alchemy.

The "I" can die only by transmuting desire into wisdom and love.

The truth comes into us only when the "I" dies.

The Occultists need to be careful not to fall into paranoia.

The delirium of paranoids is very dangerous.

Hitler was a paranoid. The Quixote of Cervantes is an example of what a paranoid is.

The delirious ideas from paranoids do not resist a logical analysis.

Many paranoids like to be inventors. Others like to be great businessmen, illustrious reformers, extraordinary prophets, etc., etc.

When we analyze their delirious ideas, we see then that they do not resist an analysis.

When their errors are shown to them, they fill themselves with supreme pain. Afterwards, they react against the person who showed them their error and accuse that person as being unjust and envious, etc., etc.

The Rosicrucian paranoid, mentioned by us in previous paragraphs, asked forgiveness of one of his critics. Afterwards, confused, he wept. When it was demanded to him to retract himself in public, he then reacted and accused his critic. This is how the paranoids are.

The Occultist, Theosophist Rosicrucians must study the sacred science without loosing their mental balance. Unfortunately, many esoterist students become paranoids.

Commonly, they feel themselves to be reincarnations of Jesus Christ, Buddha, Mohammed, Marie Antoinette, Napoleon, etc. This is how they convert themselves into Quixotes, into authentic paranoids.

This is the danger of the esoteric studies.

Many esoterists are assaulted by the delirium of grandeur; they seem to perform gigantic things, etc.

They fill themselves with malice and distrust. They believe that the whole world is bewitching them. They slander others by accusing them of being black magicians, etc., etc.

This is what a Theosophist Occultist paranoid is.

The paranoid, who did not study esoteric doctrines, thinks that he descends from Napoleon or from some Count or very famous Sage.

He assumes that he is a superman. He believes himself to be a great businessman, etc., etc.

In Mexico, we knew the case of a paranoid who assassinated many women.

Finally, when they discovered that he assassinated his fiancée, the daughter of a lawyer, he was caught and put in jail. That paranoid was burying his victims in the garden of his home.

He was affirming in the penitentiary that he only needed another victim in order to find the secret with which the human being can mock death and not ever die.

This is how the paranoids are: very intelligent and dangerous people.

According to clinical criteria, many paranoids who live normally and who are not dangerous exist. However, among them exist psychopaths who are terribly dangerous!

Commonly, the paranoid is essentially malicious and distrustful.

The paranoids are so sly that they even cheat the psychiatrists themselves.

The paranoiac constellation has many degrees.

The most socially dangerous paranoiac psychosis is the one that deprives some of these individuals of rationalism.

Consequently, when they become demented, they commit the most terrible crimes.

Chapter 30

Pedagogic Psychotherapy

Two types of criminal authors exist. The first ones are those who induce others into delinquency by means of hypnotism, spiritualism, intimidation, coaction, witchcraft, psychological constriction, etc., etc. These are the mediate authors.

The second ones are the immediate authors, those who commit the concrete crime, the factual situations, the criminal situational reactions, etc., etc.

We, the partisans of expanded psychiatry, expanded with Theosophical and Rosicrucian matters, believe that criminology is a very profound science.

Adler, Jung, and Freud have given onto psychiatry the A, B, C's of scientific criminology.

The penal code is not criminology. The penal code is only a human covenant in order to defend themselves from society.

The satyrs, for instance, are criminals even if they are not enclosed within a jail.

The endocrine-pathologies conduce to crime; nonetheless, the penal code has nothing to do with it.

Eroticism, accompanied by personal pain, is related with the instinct of power and with the sexual instinct. This is masochism. The sadist inflicts pain to his/her sexual partner in order to feel pleasure.

Those forms of sexual perversion constitute that which is called "Algolagnia."

The instinct of power and the sexual instinct are related with the diencephalon and the gray cerebral nucleus that control their manifestations.

Anger, the origin of too many bloody cases, corresponds to the instinct of power.

Love is related with the sexual glands. How many times both love and anger unite, mix, and mutually condition themselves until becoming crime!

Love and anger, sexual instinct, and instinct of power have their plusses and minuses in the biorhythm of our glands of internal secretion. We recommend the book *Biorhythm* by Dr. Krumm-Heller.

Love and anger have their mutual transferences and their most capricious psychic combinations.

Traumas and nervous impressions disturb many times the functions of the Cerebrospinal Nervous System and the functions of the Grand Sympathetic Nervous System, as well as the glands of internal secretion.

The sexual psychopathic personality has, for instance, very complex origins. The deviation of the sexual instinct and the instinct of power originates psychopathic, schizoid, and compulsive personalities of an infinite variety.

The sadists and masochists are the best example of what the deviation of the sexual instincts and the instincts of power signifies. The sadomasochists commit the bloodiest crimes that overwhelm because of their monstrosity.

Fetishism, with its black masses and witchcraft, form part of this criminal constellation.

Nevertheless, one is overwhelmed when one sees the judges laughing while in front of witchcraft with its "embos" and fetishism.

On a certain occasion, a sick individual presented himself before the Public Ministry. He came to place a complaint against his lover who he thought was bewitching him. He was exhibiting, as a *corpus delicti*, a doll filled with pins. Of course, the authorities laughed at the denouncer, and in order to be rid of him for that moment, they came up with a sophism of distraction, promising to arrest such a woman.

When that man left the office of the Public Ministry, an employee, while laughing, took away the pins from the doll and afterwards he hurled the "embo" into a water pot.

The next day, the man full of happiness and health, presented himself again before the authorities.

The man gave thanks onto the authorities, since he firmly believed that they had cured him. He was feeling himself completely sane.

What is this? What does this signify? What does the penal code state about this?

The penal code does not understand anything about this. Onto the science of criminology corresponds the study of the scientific part of fetishism and witchcraft.

It is impossible to laugh before demonstrated facts. To laugh about the "embos" in this epoch of radioactivity and in instants in which we are studying atomic physics, becomes, indeed, stubborn and absurd.

The former case that we narrated could be included in psychobiology.

The employee who took away the pins from the "embo" and afterwards hurled it into the water pot was, indeed, the doctor of that sick man.

The imagination of that man's lover, exalted by the pins of that doll, is what hurt that man.

A psychobiologic, energetic and subtle relation existed between the "embo" and the sick man. These subtle energies are as real as the waves of a radio or as the emanations of radium and cobalt.

The employee who took away the pins from the doll and hurled it into the water altered the instrument of torture, thus he cured the sick man. The employee was the doctor of the sick man.

It is necessary to awaken clairvoyance in order to study psychobiology in depth, to study it profoundly in its basis.

We need to transcend the barbaric law of retaliation and to study criminology under the light of expanded psychiatry.

It is necessary to take into account and to study the hereditary "I," the unconscious "I," the infraconscious "I," the subconscious "I," the epileptic "I," the phenotypic "I," etc., etc.

It is necessary to profoundly explore the "I" within the depths of the mind. Thereafter, to organize a transcendental psychotherapy in order to cure those unhappy delinquents.

The law of retaliation does not reform anybody. Pain is useless.

We need psychotherapy.

It is necessary to study the syndromes or psychic sicknesses. The criminological diagnostics must be based on expanded psychiatry.

It is necessary to analyze the mental alterations of ourselves based on Theosophy.

It is urgent to know the Mental Body.

It is necessary to expand forensic psychiatry.

It is necessary to study, in a didactic way, psychobiology and psychopathology.

The valuable work of Lombroso and Marro is incomplete without Theosophy. The studies of criminal anthropology, perfected by Vervaeck, when applied to the purely penitentiary system, are incomplete when psychiatry very well expanded with Theosophical wisdom is not studied.

It is necessary to make a psychosomatic analysis of the delinquent.

It is urgent to know the psychophysiology of the delinquent.

It is indispensable to study the endocrine glands of the delinquent.

It is necessary to analyze the purely psychic functions of the endocrine glands of the delinquent.

Endocrinology and criminology are found intimately correlated.

It is urgent to study the nervous systems of central relation and the vegetative organs.

After all of these studies about the delinquent, we must explore in depth his psychological "I," the most profound depths of his mind.

The diagnostic and prognostic about the personality of the delinquent are exact when we know the Theosophy and Rosicrucian subject matter.

Any science is incomplete when one does not know the occult wisdom, that is to say, Gnosis.

The diagnostic and prognostic about the delinquent must be exact; otherwise, the law of retaliation will continue.

The penitentiaries must be converted into psychiatric clinics, hospitals, universities, schools, workshops, agriculture farms, etc.

Psychotherapy is a polyphase system.

Each delinquent needs his own specialized professors.

The pedagogic corrective treatment, the pedagogic psychotherapy, must be headed by psychiatrists who truly have studied Theosophy, Rosicrucianism, Hermeticism, Yogic Philosophy, etc.; that is to say, they must be Gnostics.

The materialist psychiatrists do not achieve the reformation of delinquents. They are an absolute failure.

Materialism already failed in Soviet Russia. It is demonstrated by the evident fact that fifteen million Muslims are living within the heart of Russia.

Practically, only a few fanatics of the Creole materialism have remained who still live, in this day and age, as if this was the 18th century.

Good music, conferences, educative and highly spiritual movies, baths, hiking, a sexually healthy life, etc., etc. can reform and cure delinquents.

The law of retaliation has routinely failed.

Now we need corrective psychotherapy.

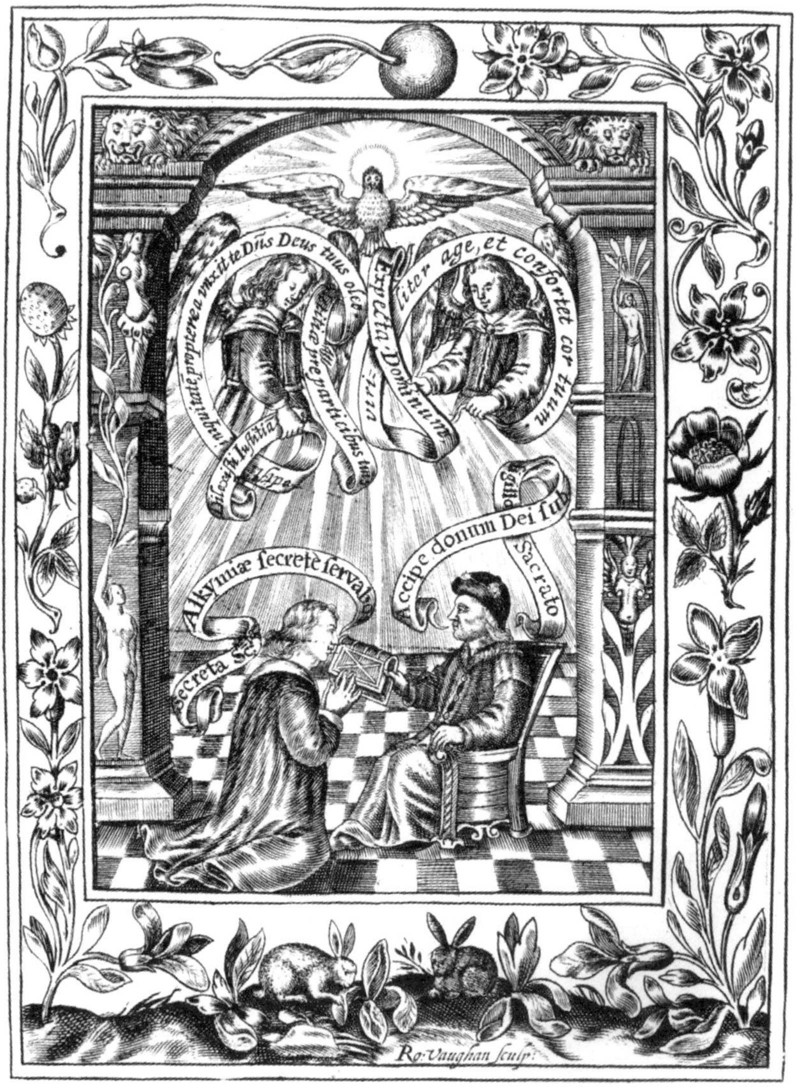

propterea vnxit te Dn̄s Deus tuus oleo
lætitiæ præ participibus tuis
Dilexisti Iustitiam
Expecta Dominum
liter age, et confortet cor tuum
Alkymiæ secretè servabo
secreta &c.
Accipe donum Dei sub
sigillo Sacrato
Ro: Vaughan sculp:

Conclusions

Endocriminology is a science that is still in an embryonic state.

Criminology is found stagnated by materialistic science.

The powers of clairvoyance, clairaudience, intuition, telepathy, omniscience, etc., etc. are found in a latent state within the endocrine glands.

The mistaken use of powers is criminal.

Ignorance is the cause of the evil use of psychic powers.

Psychiatry, expanded with Theosophical and Rosicrucian matters, will take criminology from the stagnant state in which it is found.

The penal code must be reformed with arrangements based on scientific criminology.

Psychobiology without Theosophy is like a garden without water.

Every esoterist student must have discipline and intellectual culture.

The occultist without discipline and intellectual culture converts himself into a delinquent.

The upright use of powers is a blessing for the whole world.

The unjust use of powers is a damnation for the whole world.

The ignoramus who wants to educe and develop the psychic powers that are latent in the glands of internal secretion is like a child who wants to play with dynamite.

The occultist without intellectual culture converts himself into a delinquent.

This book is a codex of scientific ethics for all the Rosicrucian Gnostics, yogis, occultists, spiritualists, etc., etc.

The esoterist who studies and accepts this book as a codex of scientific ethics will not fall into the abyss of delinquency.

This book opens a new field of investigations for psychiatry and criminology.

Index

N

O

Q

R

T

Books by the Same Author

Aquarian Message
Aztec Christic Magic
Book of the Dead
Book of the Virgin of Carmen
Buddha's Necklace
Christ Will
Christmas Messages (various)
Cosmic Ships
Cosmic Teachings of a Lama
Didactic Self-Knowledge
Dream Yoga (collected writings)
Elimination of Satan's Tail
Esoteric Course of Runic Magic
Esoteric Treatise of Hermetic Astrology
Esoteric Treatise of Theurgy
Fundamental Education
Fundamental Notions of Endocrinology
Gnostic Anthropology
Gnostic Catechism
The Great Rebellion
Greater Mysteries
Igneous Rose
The Initiatic Path in the Arcana of Tarot and Kabbalah
Introduction to Gnosis
Kabbalah of the Mayan Mysteries
Lamasery Exercises
Logos Mantra Theurgy
Manual of Practical Magic
Mysteries of Fire: Kundalini Yoga
Mystery of the Golden Blossom
Occult Medicine & Practical Magic
Parsifal Unveiled
The Perfect Matrimony
Pistis Sophia Unveiled
Revolution of Beelzebub
Revolution of the Dialectic
Revolutionary Psychology
Secret Doctrine of Anahuac
Three Mountains
Transmutation of Sexual Energy
Treatise of Sexual Alchemy
Yellow Book
Yes, There is Hell, a Devil, and Karma
Zodiacal Course
150 Answers from Master Samael Aun Weor

To learn more about Gnosis, visit gnosticteachings.org.

Thelema Press is a non-profit publisher dedicated to spreading the sacred universal doctrine to suffering humanity. All of our works are made possible by the kindness and generosity of sponsors. If you would like to make a tax-deductible donation, you may send it to the address below, or visit our website for other alternatives. If you would like to sponsor the publication of a book, please contact us at 212-501-6106 or help@gnosticteachings.org.

Thelema Press
PMB 192, 18645 SW Farmington Rd., Aloha OR 97007 USA
Phone: 212-501-6106 · Fax: 212-501-1676

Visit us online at:
gnosticteachings.org
gnosticradio.org
gnosticschool.org
gnosticstore.org
gnosticvideos.org